PRAISE FOR
CHEF ANI PHYO and SMARTMONKEY FOODS:

"The recipes are scrumptious, the fare is healthy, fresh. The facts are truly interesting. A breath of fresh air."

—Ingrid Newkirk, founder of PETA

"Ani Phyo's Raw Food Kitchen is a lovely addition to any home and kitchen. By using the recipes in this book you will learn how and why raw food is the coolest trend to emerge out of California since surfing."

—David Wolfe, founder of www.sunfood.com, author of *The Sunfood Diet Success System, Eating for Beauty,* and *Naked Chocolate*

"With beautiful photography and delicious easy-to-follow healthy recipes, *Ani's Raw Food Kitchen* is an essential new addition to my library and kitchen!"

—Robert Cheeke, Founder/President, Vegan Bodybuilding and Fitness

"Phyo shows how to create more complex flavor harmonies. Nutmeats of all sorts serve as a basis of many recipes, offering a spectrum of uses from cheese substitutions to pie crusts."

—Booklist

"*Ani's Raw Food Kitchen* will surprise you with recipes that somehow seem very familiar even if you've never eaten them before. Ani's. . . ultra-busy just like the rest of us, so most of her advice is easy to implement and her recipes are often quick to prepare."

—boingboing.net

"Raw foods have become very popular among Hollywood's film industry—and I'm the man who feeds them. I will definitely keep SmartMonkey Food's Walnut Cranberry Squash Rice in my rotation. The response to Ani's raw rice on set [*Pirates of the Caribbean III*] was overwhelming, and the director of the film thinks it rocks."

—Teddy Yonenaka, Phat Teddy's Green Craft Service

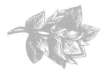

ani phyo is an executive chef overseeing everything created by SmartMonkey Foods, the premier resource for vegan, raw, and living cuisine that's full of flavor, design, and creativity and packed full of fresh local organics. She is a sought-after speaker and educator on the topics of health, fitness, and overall well-being. Visit her at www.aniphyo.com.

ani's raw
food kitchen

Also by Ani Phyo:

*Return on Design: Smarter
Web Design That Works*

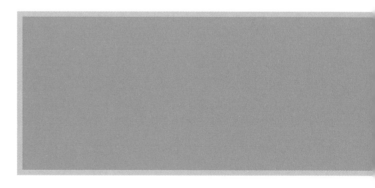

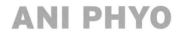

ANI PHYO

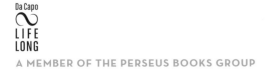

ani's raw
food kitchen

Easy, Delectable Living Foods Recipes

Da Capo
∞
LIFE
LONG

A MEMBER OF THE PERSEUS BOOKS GROUP

Copyright © 2007 by Ani Phyo
Photographs by:
Ede Schweizer (California: cover, lifestyle, kitchen prep, and recipes)
Duc Nguyen (Ingredients: vegetables and fruits)
Jim Yeager (Portland: farmers market, Bagdad Theatre, Stumpton Café)
Icon illustrations by Antonio Sanchez

Cataloging-in-Publication data for this book is available from the Library of Congress.

ISBN-13: 978-1-60094-000-2

Published by Da Capo Press
A Member of the Perseus Books Group
www.dacapopress.com

Da Capo Press books are available at special discounts for bulk purchases in the U.S. by corporations, institutions, and other organizations. For more information, please contact the Special Markets Department at the Perseus Books Group, 2300 Chestnut Street, Suite 200, Philadelphia, PA, 19103, or call (800) 255-1514, or e-mail special.markets@perseusbooks.com.

This book is dedicated to Ede Schweizer.

Thank you for shining so brightly, for

inspiring me, for dreaming with me, for

believing in me, and for jumping in to

save the day again and again.

You're my hero.

contents

introduction   1

    Fresh Living Cuisine   8

    Here's to Your Health   12

    Kitchen Tools for Raw Living Foods   15

    Going to the Market   17

    Shopping Checklist   25

    Using This Book   36

1 drinks for radiance   41

    Smoothies   46

        Very Blueberry   46

        Mango Lassi   47

        Carob Strawberry Bliss   47

        Piña Colada   48

        Pear Frosty   48

        Black Sesame Jewel   49

    Shake It Up   50

        Brazilian Carob Shake   50

        Vanilla Coconut Shake   50

        Strawberry Coconut Shake   51

        Cherry Malt   51

        Peachy Kream   52

        Fuzzy Navel   52

        Carob Almond Decadence   53

        Almond Nog   53

        Blue-Green Power   54

Mylks   54
    Vanilla Mylk   55
    Chocolate Mylk   56
    Cinnamon Banana Buttermylk   56
    Yum Yum Mylk   57
    Made in Mexico Mylk   57
    Chocolate-Hazelnut Mylk   58
    Beautifying Pumpkin Mylk   58
    Cashew Banana Mylk   59
    Praline Mylk   59

Juice   60
    Green Machine   60

2 breakfast of champions   63

Cereals   66
    Buckwheat Crispies   66
    Goji Berry Sunshine Cereal   67
    Good Morning Muesli   68
    Nirvana Hemp Muesli   68
    Almond Cinnamon Oatmeal   69
    Banana Raisin Oatmeal   69
    SmartMonkey Bar Oatmeal   71
    SmartMonkey Bar Cereal   71

Puddings   72
    Carob Pudding   73
    Cacao Pudding   73
    Cashew Coconut Pudding   73
    Luscious Lemon Pudding   74
    Fruit Parfait   75
    Crepe Kream Stack   76

Inspired by Pancakes   77
    Coconut Breakfast Cakes   78

Syrups   79
    Berry-licious Syrup   79
    Orange Vanilla Syrup   79
    Vanilla Syrup   79

Butters   80
    Olive Butter   80
    Coconut Butter   80

Chicken-Friendly Scrambles   81
    Love-the-Chicks Pâté   81
    Garden Scramble   82
    Spanish Scramble   82
    Asian Scramble   83

3 fresh salads and simple dressings

                                              85

Salads   92
    Shaved Fennel with Blood Oranges, Poppy Seeds,   93
      and Micro Greens
    Cabbage Kale Slaw in Simple Greek Dressing   94
    Confetti Salad in Orange-Cucumber Dressing   95
    Spring Herb Rainbow in Creamy Curry Dressing   96
    Evergreen Salad in Sunflower Thyme Marinade   97
    Asian Greens Salad with Super Asian Dressing   98
    Thai Salad Mix with Kaffir Lime Leaf Dressing   99
    Wilted Spinach Salad with Marinated Onions   100
      in Mustard Seed Dressing
    Arugula with Golden Beets and Walnuts   101
      in Orange Miso Dressing
    Spinach Salad with Persimmons and Spiced Pecans   102
      in Shallot Lemon Dressing
    Wakame Hemp Power Slaw   103
    Black Sesame Asian Slaw with Ginger Cashew Mayo   105

4 soups and sauces to tickle your tongue

                                              107

Nourishing Soups   115
    Heirloom Tomato Gazpacho   115
    Garlic Walnut Soup   116
    Creamy Portabello Bisque   117
    Japanese Miso-Shiitake Soup   118
    Tomato Basil Bisque   120
    Lemon Fennel Soup   121
    Sweet Corn Chowder   122

Thailand Tom Kha Gai 123
Spicy Kream of Avocado Soup 124
Home-Style Minestrone Soup 125

Savory Sauces and Dips 126
Sun-Dried Tomato Marinara 126
Garlic Cashew Aïoli 127
Miso Gravy 127
Kreamy Almond Yogurt 128
Tzaziki—Cucumbers in Yogurt 129
Sun-Dried Tomato Catsup 129
Hot Mustard Sauce 130

5 accompaniments and sides 133
Coconut Chutney 138
Walnut Cranberry Squash "Rice" 140
Mexican Squash "Rice" 142
Thai-Style Cucumbers 142
Brazil-Broccoli Mash 143
Cauliflower Miso Mash 143
Indian-Spiced Cashews 144
Sweet Spiced Pecans 145
Mediterranean Dolmas 146
Cashew Sour Kream and Chives 147
Sun-Dried Tomato Hummus (Bean-Free) 148
Black Olive Hummus (Bean-Free) 149
Pistachio Pesto 150
Rosemary Guacamole 150
Red Pepper Corn Salsa 151
Cashew Garlic Parmesan Sprinkle 151
Asparagus with Cheezy Sauce 152
Black Sesame Sunflower Bread 153
Black Sesame Sunflower Croutons 154
Taco Nut Meat 154
Homemade Black Olive Tapenade 155

6 scrumptious cheezes and pâtés 157

Cheezes 160
Italian Pizza Cheeze 161

Black Pepper Cheeze 161
Crushed Red Pepper–Crusted Cheeze Patty 162
Sun-Dried Tomato Cheeze 162
Herb-Crusted Cheese Patty 163
Ricotta Cheeze 163
Sunny Dill Cheeze 164
Baja Cheeze 164
Oregano Ricotta 165
Nacho Cheeze 165

Pâtés 166
Save-the-Tuna Pâté 166
Ginger Almond Pâté 167
Garden Pâté 167

7 moreish mains

169

Wrap and Roll 176
Italian Herb Collard Wrap 177
Thai Spring Rolls with Dipping Sauce 178
Save-the-Tuna Wrap 179
Save-the-Tuna Roll 180
Ginger Almond Nori Roll 181

Better Than Pastas 182
Fettuccini Squash Noodles in Alfredo Sauce 182
Angel-Hair Squash Pasta in Pesto Sauce 183
Angel-Hair Squash Noodles in Sun-Dried Tomato Marinara 184
Italian Rawzania 185
Pad Thai Noodles in Almond Kaffir Sauce 186
Mushroom Risotto with White Truffle–Infused Olive Oil 188

More Main Dishes That Make You Sing 189
Baja Cheeze Burrito with Taco Nut Meat 189
and Red Pepper Corn Salsa
Polenta with Mushroom Ragout 190
Stuffed Anaheim Chiles with Mole Sauce 192
Save-the-Salmon Patties with Hollandaise Sauce 193
Sun Burgers on Black Sesame Sunflower Bread 194
with Sun-Dried Tomato Catsup

Marinated Portabello Steak and Brazil-Broccoli Mash   196
    with Mushroom Gravy
Pizza with Sun-Dried Tomatoes, Black Olives,   197
    and Fresh Italian Herbs

8   decadent desserts

    199

Dessert Soups   207
    Strawberry Kream Swirl   207
    Blueberry Soup with Cashew Kream   208
    Fuzzy Navel con Kream   209

Pies and Cobblers   210
    All-American Apple Pie   211
    Pecan Chai Pie on Cashew Crust   212
    Persimmon Pie   213
    Summer Berry Cobbler   214
    Fresh Mango Cobbler   215
    Fresh Mission Fig and Pear Tart   216
    Coconut Cream Pie with Carob Fudge on Brownie Crust   217
    Autumn Pumpkin Pie   218

Cakes   219
    Deep Forest Carob Cake with Fudge Frosting   219
    Coconut Snow Cake   220
    Carrot Cake with Kream Cheeze Frosting   222
    The Real Cheezecake   223
    Florida Orange-Spice Bars   224
    Carob Crunch Torte   226
    Lemon Coconut Bars   227
    Dreaming About Donut Holes   228

Icey Kreams   229
    Hazelnut Gelato   229
    Vanilla Macadamia Ice Kream   230
    Puckering Lemon Mint Ice   230
    Fresh Apricot Sorbet   231

Sweet Sauces   232
    Carob Sauce   232
    Raspberry Sauce   233
    Berry Compote   233

9 kanga's dandy dog food   235

    Kanga's Favorite Pâté   240
    Kanga Dog Treats   241
    Black Sesame Sunflower Dog Biscuits   242

Thanks   243
Index   245

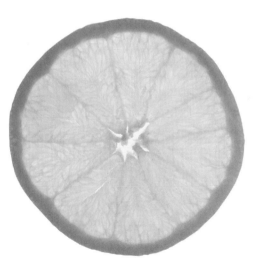

Oranges are perfectly packaged by
Mother Nature as a great travel snack.

This book is the green living resource for busy, health-conscious people who want to eat more fresh organic living foods that are fast and easy to make, delicious and nutritious to enjoy.

introduction

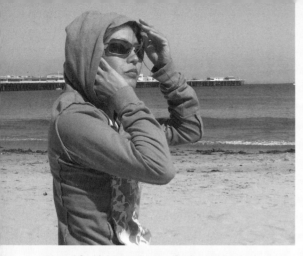

Good food can make you feel more lively, look better, and perform at your best.

I'VE ALWAYS BEEN a connoisseur of flavorful world cuisine. And while my interest in healthy eating has changed the way my kitchen looks (ovens are so overrated), my passion for great taste has never faded.

What's the secret to great taste? Simplicity. Just like a work of art, you need to know when to stop adding ingredients and realize a dish is done. Of course, that's not always so easy to do. Especially when you have an array of seasonal herbs and produce to choose from.

The local farmers' market is my daily source for inspiration. Whatever produce is the ripest in the morning is what you'll find on my table that afternoon. It has to be organic and it has to be fresh. If you haven't been to a farmers' market before, try visiting one before planning your next menu. You'll find they're full of fresh ideas.

In a way, you could say this book is like a farmers' market in itself. Just take a leisurely stroll through the pages. You'll discover it has a lot to offer, from healthy-lifestyle tips—like living garbage-free, buying seasonally and locally, and using natural cleansers and beauty products—to innovative meals that are easy to prepare.

And by "easy to prepare," I mean exactly that. Prep time for these recipes is minimal, and all the ingredients can be found at your local street market or grocery store. My main goal is to get you into the kitchen so that you can start enjoying these natural flavors today— fresh cuisine mixed with a little urban flair. I realize a 100 percent raw diet may be too extreme for some. This isn't a "raw or nothing" book. Everyone can benefit from enjoying more whole organic fresh foods, and these recipes will help you add more goodness into any diet. Sound yummy to you? Great. Let's eat.

MY PATH TO LIVE FOODS

I've come full circle, back to the way I was raised. I remember tending to my family's organic garden as a child, and watching my dad bite into a red pepper like it was an apple. I thought this was so unsophisticated, something carried over from the *old* country.

Once again, I'm fueling myself with fresh, organic, uncooked whole fruits, vegetables, herbs, spices, nuts, and seeds. This time I'm on a mission to show everyone that nutritious is delicious. The "old days" of unappealing health foods like mud-sludge vegetable juices to be gulped down while plugging my nose have now evolved into delicious and artful cuisine. The recipes in this book need no excuses to be eaten, but are instead enjoyed as simply yummy food. It's all about the flavor and feeling great.

I've spent many years searching out what foods maintain a high degree of health but still mesh well with my urban lifestyle. Traveling the world, I've discovered that it's obvious humans

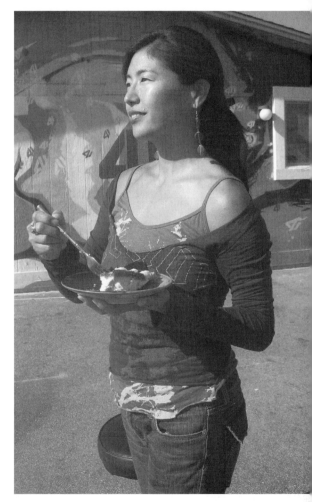

I love sunshine, outdoor adventures, and yummy desserts.

can live eating almost anything. I believe eating living foods is the optimal way to fuel our bodies, connect with our food source to ensure its high quality, and enjoy every last bite.

Having studied nutrition for more than a couple of decades, I had to figure out how to fuel my body for optimal performance to enhance my life and avoid getting sick. I was stoked to discover gourmet living foods at Juliano's Raw Restaurant in San Francisco. It tasted so delicious, unlike the boring raw foods I'd been raised on. I quickly noticed I couldn't sleep after a raw dinner. I had so much energy, mental clarity, and focus, I found I could efficiently crank out tons of work.

Soon I began consulting for studios in Los Angeles. Spending more and more time in corporate buildings, it broke my heart each day to see so many people repeatedly using Styrofoam cups to drink one cup of water, then throwing it away. There were no recycling programs in place. And my office buildings were cooled to uncomfortably cold temperatures when it was over a hundred degrees outside. Employees would wear winter jackets and work at their desks with blankets over their shoulders. This waste of energy and resources was too much for me to take.

So I decided to trade in my design career for one in which I can help others learn about health, nutrition, getting the most out of life, and treading lightly on our planet for our children's future. At the same time, I'm showing people how to find the best, most nutritious ingredients to fuel their bodies.

The seeds for SmartMonkey Foods were planted in Santa Monica, California. For two years I worked

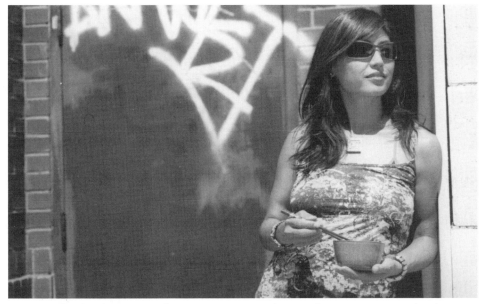

I carry my food with me everywhere I go. As a sun seeker, I make sure to enjoy my lunch outside every day.

alongside Juliano, who many credit as ushering raw into its current "vogue." He taught me everything he knew about raw-food cuisine, and I guzzled it down like a fresh smoothie.

Soon I began developing recipes of my own and contributing them to Juliano's menu. And the dishes were a hit. I found myself hosting raw-food events of my own around the city. The name SmartMonkey Foods became synonymous with great food, organic wines, stimulating conversation, and incredible music.

The events were held in huge, open warehouses where people could participate in making the food. These weekly gourmet dinners became one of the hottest tickets in town, attracting a great range of people, from artists and musicians to well-known actors. Soon people began asking me to cater weeklong menus for pickup at the beginning of the week. I started packaging sauces, dressings, cheezes, pâtés, soups, breads, and desserts. The foods were designed to travel well and were quick to assemble. It was the beginning of the SmartMonkey Foods line.

SMART
MONKEY
FOODS™
SMARTMONKEYFOODS.com

Kanga loves walking to the co-op with me. She has her own backpack and even helps me carry groceries home sometimes. Today we're joined by the lovely SmartMonkey Heather Butler.

It was hard to imagine life could get any better. That is, until I discovered a city called Portland, Oregon. It's a city made up of artists, musicians, and small, locally owned businesses. Plus, it has a great public transit system, many green businesses, bike lanes on most roads, and an abundance of clean air and water.

Today I think of the entire West Coast as my home, especially Southern and Northern California and Portland, Oregon. I continue to teach classes on live-food nutrition and preparation, and host dinners and special events—all of which keep growing in popularity. SmartMonkey Foods is all about recipes that balance flavor, nutrition, and well-being—something everyone can appreciate. You are what you eat. So why not eat healthy?

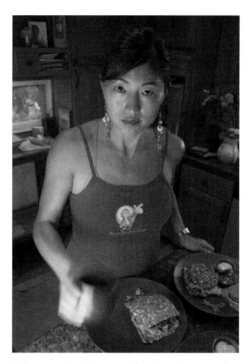

Cheers, a toast to good food!

WEST COAST RAW

I do a lot of work throughout the West Coast and have found *raw* means different things in different regions. The folks in Southern California turn to raw living foods for weight loss and antiaging benefits. In Northern California, folks turn to raw living foods for health reasons. And in the Pacific Northwest, I find people interested in live foods for its physical performance benefits, because the people are outdoorsy and active. Along the entire West Coast, everyone loves the green living aspects that come along with eating this way.

fresh living cuisine

WHAT ARE "LIVING FOODS"?

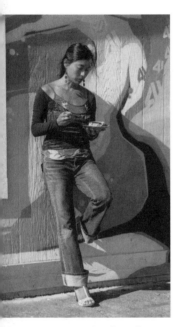

Organic foods in their most natural, uncooked state are packed full of taste, nutrients, and enzymes.

I call unheated fresh foods "living foods." You might also hear it called "life food" or "live food." It's always organic, fresh as can be, and I never heat anything above 104ºF, if at all. This is a lower temperature than others may choose, but I figure water gets painful to the touch above 104ºF, so it must be doing damage to my cells and killing enzymes.

Living foods are full of enzyme activity. Enzymes help you digest food and are the catalysts for every metabolic reaction in your body. Without these enzymes, there can be no cell division, energy production, or brain activity.

I define "living" and "raw" foods differently. Water is the basis of all life. Some foods may be "raw," but have less enzyme activity than if they were "living." For example, a raw cracker that's overly dehydrated lacks water. It may have been low-heat processed, but I sometimes find it hard to digest. Here's another illustration, this one from nature: a nut or seed is eaten by a bird or animal, then dropped into the moist soil. The seed or nut begins to germinate, to create new life. This soaked and germinated nut is very different from a dormant unsoaked nut that's just raw—it's living.

Only uncooked and unprocessed foods can provide us with the full range of vitamins, minerals, enzymes, oxygen, fiber, and other nutrients our bodies require to run like a well-oiled machine. Living foods are the key to health and nutrition, and in turn, fuel optimal performance.

FRESH ORGANICS FOR BODY, MIND, AND SPIRIT

OXYGEN is one of our most important nutrients. In urban centers with fewer trees and more pollution, there's less oxygen. Plus, we've got the highest levels in history of CO_2 in our air today, due to pollution and global warming.

Oxygen's more available in uncooked food. Fresh fruit and vegetables are up to 90 percent water and 60 percent oxygen. It's already been proven that cancer can't exist in highly oxygenated environments!

Living foods give life. Put an orange or avocado into the earth, and a tree or plant will grow from it. Many health experts believe living and raw foods are the key to good health and longevity.

WATER is the basis of all life. Our blood is more than 80 percent water, and our liver is 96 percent water. Water from fresh fruits and vegetables helps our body flush out toxins we're exposed to in our air, processed or nonorganic foods, and things we touch.

FIBER acts like a broom sweeping through the body, and water is the hose that washes away impurities. Think of our bodies as finely tuned machines, and living vegan foods burn cleaner than any other fuel. It's the rocket fuel for your body.

The human body is amazingly able to run on the lowest grade fuel, but imagine how much that takes away from the overall life of the vehicle. Eating as nature intended helps keep you fit, healthy, and vibrant. Once you begin incorporating living foods into your diet, you'll notice an increase in mental clarity and focus and a more positive outlook on life.

MINDFULNESS of what I choose to put into my body and the businesses I support with my dollars makes me feel good about myself. Knowing no animals were harmed while doing good for my health and the planet is good karma. You'll see a huge decrease in the amount of garbage in your kitchen with the more fresh living foods you enjoy. A lot of the garbage we generate comes from packaging from processed foods; eating fresh ingredients helps cut down on the amount of waste we create.

LIFE force to me is simply energy. So eating the freshest foods with the most life force raises my energy levels.

ENZYMES rejuvenate our bodies. They carry nutrients to the cellular level, keeping cells clean and healthy. Our body regenerates entirely new cells every seven years. This means you can regenerate a more beautiful and vibrant body.

FRESH ORGANICS = HEALTHY PEOPLE + HEALTHY PLANET

Organic foods are more nutritious and kinder to the planet than conventionally grown foods. They contain more vitamins and minerals, and more nutrition per spoonful

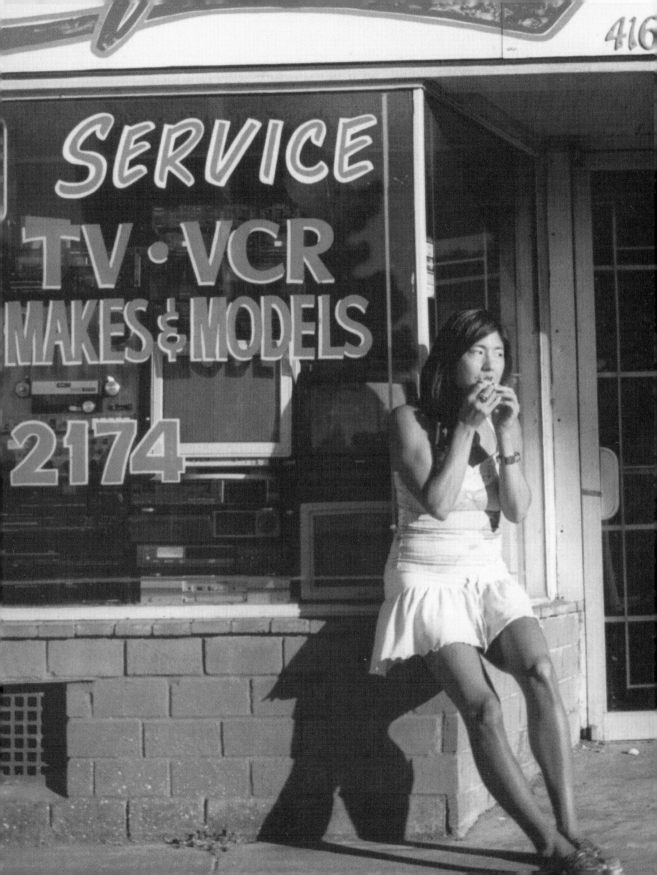

because they're farmed on mineral-rich soils. Organics don't use chemicals like pesticides or fertilizers—and that's healthier for our bodies. These chemicals aren't contaminating the earth's water supply, either.

Pesticides and herbicides reduce soil nutrients and kill all the beneficial organisms in the soil. What you end up with is dead dirt, or infertile, barren soil that's unusable for growing. Once chemicals are in the land, they're hard to clean up and remove. And when crops are sprayed, the wind can carry particles of pesticides hundreds of miles. Rain washes pesticides and chemicals into our lakes, rivers, and groundwater, poisoning their inhabitants and all that drink or eat from them, including us!

here's to your health

BENEFITS OF EATING FRESH LIVE FOODS

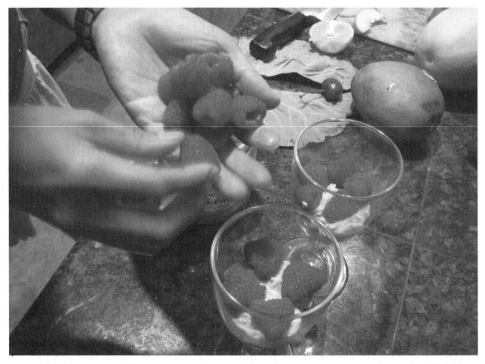

Eating freshly prepared fruits, nuts, and vegetables allows everyone to embrace healthful living while at the same time keeping the balance of nature in mind. This exciting approach to food preparation opens the door to fresh new ways of celebrating flavor and texture.

As a kid, I thought anything "good for me" would taste awful. This was mostly because my mom would throw a bunch of different veggies into the often-earthy, brown morning juice we were forced to drink before school. More proved not to mean better. Today I've come to love combining just a few fresh vegetables for their vibrant flavor, color, and texture.

I eat raw and living foods to maintain the mental clarity I've discovered through eating this way. I haven't had the flu or a cold in over eight years. And when I first began eating 100 percent fresh living foods, I lost fifteen pounds, noticed I didn't create any garbage in my kitchen anymore, and had boundless energy. I just love the way this food makes me feel.

FEED YOUR BODY WHAT IT NEEDS

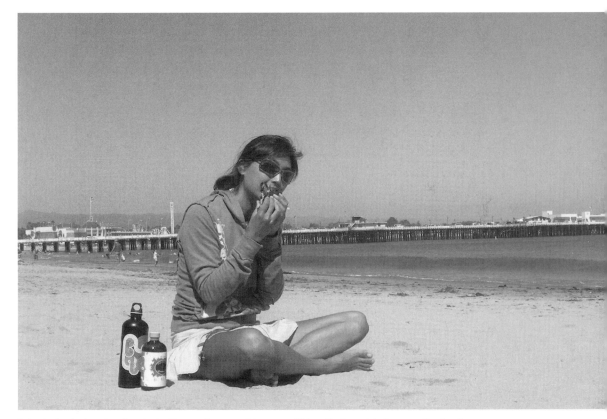

I don't think there's a book that's ever been written, or will be, that could give you the best insight into what you should be eating. You're an expert on what your body needs to perform at its best. Be your own nutritionist; discover what foods make your body purr.

LIVING GREEN, EVEN IN URBAN PLACES

It doesn't get much better than sharing a menu of vibrant foods with friends and family. Even though most of the people in my life don't share my level of passion about healthy foods, they still understand the benefits of living foods and have incorporated many of my recipes into their daily routines. You don't need to be on a 100 percent living-foods diet to feel the benefits. And the idea of eating tons of protein is an American myth. You can get all the nutrients you need from fresh living foods.

If you're not yet ready to be sporting a bio-diesel vehicle, you can always contribute by choosing renewable energy generated from the sun, wind, and biomass as a low-cost way to offset pollution from electricity usage. Green energy companies are helping our planet by working with local energy companies to provide renewable energy options to their customers. With the price of wind energy dropping, it's surprisingly cheaper than you'd think. SmartMonkey Foods uses renewable power from wind, geothermal, and low-impact hydro for only about 8 percent more than the cost of conventional power sources.

Even in an urban environment, you can take easy steps to help the environment— literally! Drive less, take public transit, bike, or walk around town. It's also easy to compost using a worm box or a compost tumbler bin, or even composting in your neighborhood garden. You can generate your own energy with devices like solar dehydrators, crank mixers and blenders, and pedal blenders.

Of course, buying organics and buying in bulk mean living green, even in urban places. Every little bit helps.

kitchen tools for raw living foods

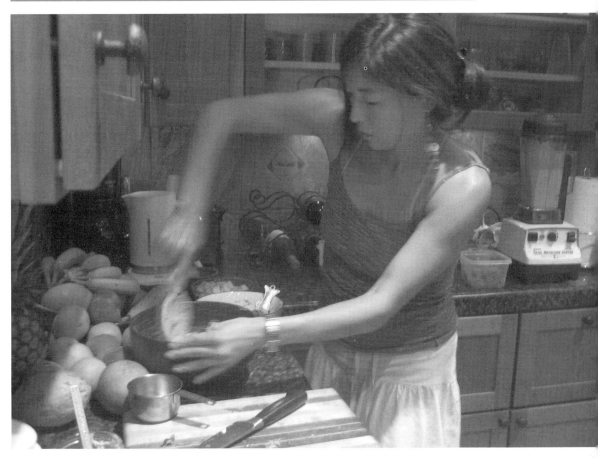

I've been known to travel with my food processor and blender in my luggage. Luckily, this kitchen came equipped with a Vita-Mix blender and food processor, so I had more space to pack clothes this trip.

KITCHEN ESSENTIALS

Two main tools to use are a food processor and blender. When helping to set up a raw kitchen, I usually start out with a food processor. You can get quality processors for about $50. I'll add in a blender for about $350–$450 later. You can find less expensive blenders to use right away, but I recommend saving up for the Vita-Mix if possible. You'll be so much happier in the long run, and it'll last your lifetime.

FOOD PROCESSOR

Food processors are used to slice, grate, chop, and puree without having to add water. One that holds at least 5 cups will probably be most useful for you.

HIGH-SPEED BLENDER

I use blenders to make liquid foods like smoothies, dressings, and soups. There are several high-quality brands of high-speed blenders on the market. Vita-Mix is my brand of choice. I've had mine for years. It's made food for thousands of people and is still going strong.

While others will work, I prefer the variable-speed model. It has a knob that allows you to gradually increase the speed so the contents don't splatter all over the place.

A high-speed blender is great because you can throw in all your ingredients and blend. I can put in an entire vanilla bean, and my Vita-Mix pulverizes the bark.

TOOLS YOU DON'T "NEED," BUT ARE FUN TO HAVE AROUND

You'll find these icons next to each recipe so you'll know what to use:

 JULIENNE PEELER   **DEHYDRATOR**

 CITRUS JUICER   **MANDOLINE SLICER**

 SPIRALIZER   **VEGETABLE JUICER**
(Saladacco or spiral slicer)

 WIRE WHISK   **ICE CREAM MAKER**

Some recipes simply require your hands and a knife

And you may want to think about getting a cutting board and knife to use just for your vegan food prep. I prefer wood or bamboo, rather than plastic, cutting boards.

going to the market

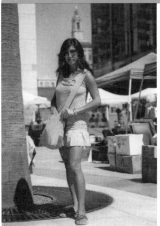

My first choice is shopping at a farmers' market or natural food store, because I prefer the selection of natural, high-quality and organic food and products. I'm a shopper who goes for quality over quantity.

AT FIRST GLANCE, natural foods and organics may seem more expensive than the regular grocery store or conventional produce. Keep in mind you actually get more for your money when buying organic fresh produce, because it's nutrient dense, without any fillers.

I think of it as investing in preventive care. Rather than paying on the back end for treatment of disease, illness, and medical bills, I'm actively preventing future illness by being as healthy as possible from the start.

My body is my temple. My body isn't a discount body. Just because something is cheap or free doesn't mean I need to eat it, especially if I know it'll do me more harm than good.

If you're shopping at a grocery store, the rule of thumb is to stay along the outside edges, where all the fresh stuff is. The middle of a store is where products can sit on shelves for a year or more. Fresh is always better.

GREEN TIP

Shop for Quality over Convenience

INSTEAD OF BUYING poor quality, disposable products because they cost less and are more convenient, opt for the more expensive, longer lasting, durable product. You'll be saving money in the long run and creating less trash.

Think about what makes a product inexpensive. How little were workers paid to work, and under what sort of conditions? And at what cost to our environment and the planet are materials available for so cheap?

FARMERS' MARKETS

By shopping at a farmers' market, you're supporting the small local organic farmer. The produce arrives super fresh, straight from the farm, usually picked just a few hours before. You'll notice how much longer this produce keeps, compared with what you'd buy at a regular grocery store.

Buying direct from farmers means bulk buying without packaging. Bringing your own bags is another way to conserve. This helps you tread lightly on our planet by using fewer resources. By supporting local farmers and businesses, your money will more likely end up being used to help your community thrive rather than helping a huge corporation expand its business.

NATURAL FOOD STORES

I like supporting community- or worker-owned food co-ops and natural food stores that strengthen the community and create less stress on the environment. Larger natural food chains like Wild Oats and Whole Foods Markets have a rigorous application process for accepting new products. They won't carry a food product with an unhealthy ingredient, or a product that's not eco-friendly, so I feel good about things I buy there.

GREEN TIP

Recycling Helps, but Reusing is Better

A LOT OF energy is used and pollution is created in the recycling process. Recycling keeps a lot of paper, glass, plastic, and aluminum out of our overflowing landfills. But if you can keep garbage out of these landfills in the first place, that's better yet.

Bring your own bags and containers when shopping. Many grocery stores will offer discounts on your purchases when you bring your own bags or containers to reuse. And cloth bags are great to leave in your car so that you'll always have them when you need them.

I ride my vintage Hawthorne to the farmers' market and fill up my basket several times a week. It's quite the social scene, and I like connecting with my friends and farmers there. Smart Monkey Kris Dyer helps me shop for our upcoming events.

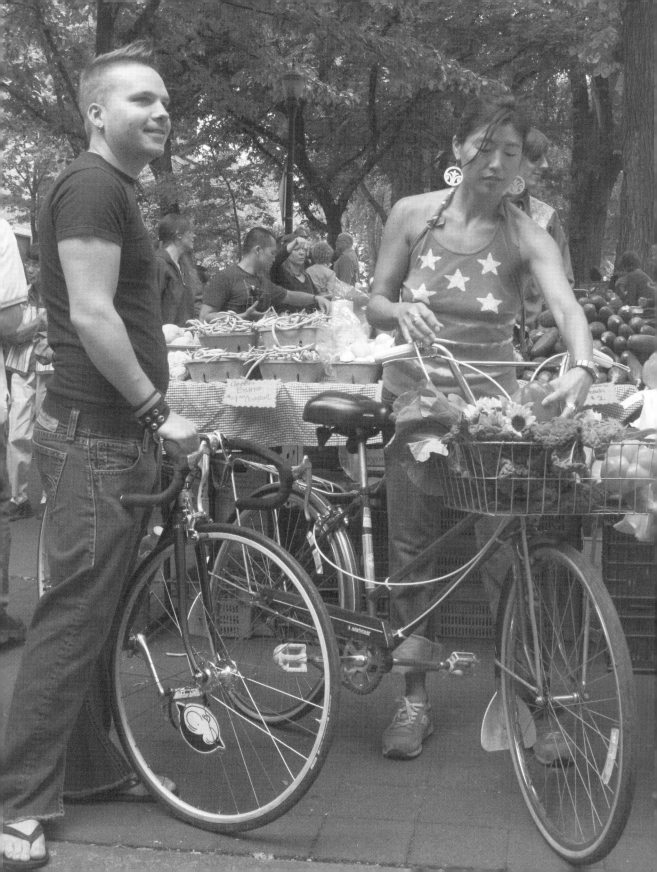

FRESH, RIPE, AND ORGANIC

Using the freshest and highest quality ingredients I can get my hands on is super important to me. This means organic, ripe, and ready to eat.

Organic produce may not look as "perfect" as conventional, but imperfections and variations are a good thing, a sign of nature. No two trees ever look identical, do they?

To avoid throwing away spoiled produce, select an amount you can use within a short time. I like to use my sense of smell to find fresh produce that is bright in color and is free of signs of spoilage, such as mold. Bacteria can thrive in the bruised areas, so avoid bruised produce and handle produce gently.

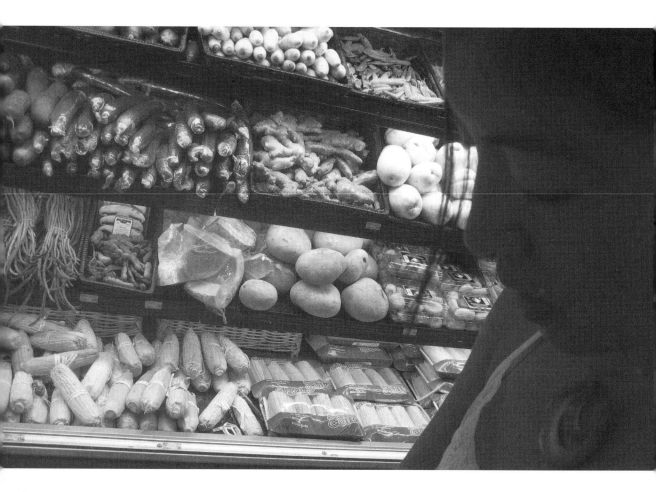

BUY LOCAL

Food tastes better and is more nutritious when it's fresh and doesn't travel as far. Buying locally saves energy and reduces carbon dioxide emissions that contribute to global warming. Most food travels an average of 1,500 miles from the farm gate to your plate by truck, boat, or plane. Buying local supports your regional economy, preserves farmland, and keeps farmers in business.

When buying locally, it's easy to eat seasonally. Keeping in sync with nature's rhythm gives us the most flavor and nutritional value when it's the most affordable.

Shopping at the farmers' markets means enjoying the freshest local seasonal produce. My good friend Duc Nguyen and I ride to the markets and enjoy connecting with the local farmers there.

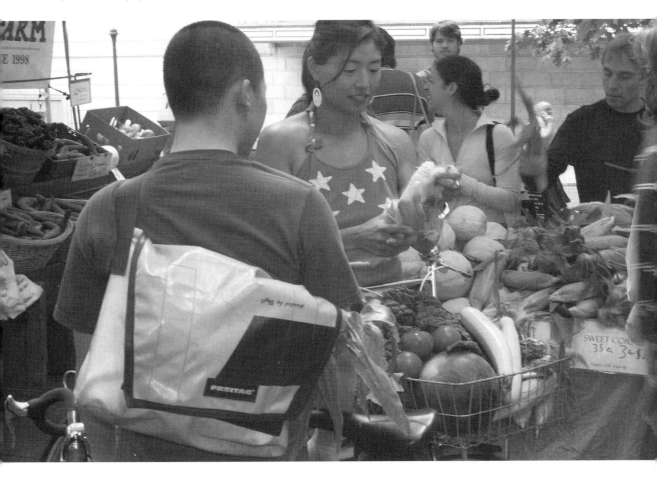

BUY SEASONAL

If you want food that's good for your health, kind to the environment, and bursting with flavor, then reconnect with the seasons. Enjoy the highest quality foods at their peak.

Seasonal food brings variety to our plates. It's important to eat a range of different foods to ensure we get all of the different nutrients we need. Besides, I like having to wait for stuff. The first blackberries in Oregon or the first persimmons in Southern California are seasonal treats to look forward to.

Growing and raising seasonal food encourages traditional agricultural methods, biodiversity, and a better environment. Plus, it promotes better-tasting food. When you see tomatoes in the store in the winter, keep in mind these aren't "natural" and by purchasing them you're compromising taste and the health of our planet.

SPRING

This is the time for tender, leafy vegetables. The green new growth that blooms in springtime should be represented by greens on your plate, including Swiss chard, spinach, romaine lettuce, and fresh herbs like parsley and basil. Also enjoy asparagus, cabbages, cauliflower, fennel, grapefruit, and navel oranges.

SUMMER

Enjoy light, cooling fruits like strawberries, pears, plums, apricots, blackberries, nectarines, peaches, limes, and melons. Vegetables like summer squash, broccoli, cauliflower, red onions, cucumber, and corn are in season now, as are spices and seasonings like peppermint and cilantro.

AUTUMN

Go for the more warming, autumn harvest foods like carrots, onions, garlic, grapes, Valencia oranges, Asian pears, and apples. Emphasize the more warming spices and seasonings like ginger, mustard seed, and peppers.

WINTER

Most root vegetables, including carrots, beets, rutabagas, onions, leeks, pumpkins, squashes, turnips, brussels sprouts, garlic, and nuts, are warming foods. Enjoy lemons, mandarins, tangerines, broccoli, and grapefruit.

WHERE DOES MY FOOD COME FROM?

Most fruits and vegetables, organic and conventional, travel an average of 1,500 miles from farm to table. This is why our foods have been bred for transport rather than taste.

Buying locally means helping to preserve diversity. Local crops are bred for flavor, not mass production. Different heirloom varieties each have their own unique flavors and carry traits allowing them to survive and adapt to new pests and changing climates.

Mainstream supermarkets bring us an abundance of foods all year round from all over the world. The modern food industry has taken away any burden of having to worry or learn about our food supply. As a result, we have sacrificed taste and nutrients. I'd rather eat a local fresh tomato than one that was picked green, gassed to redness, and shipped across the country.

I care about our environment and planet and the energy used in food production. What we choose to eat has a tremendous impact on our planet. Huge heated green-houses pump out CO_2 so we can eat out-of-season cucumbers, and mangoes are shipped to us from Guatemala in the wintertime, for example. Our fight with the seasons is accelerating climate change. Produce that's in season hasn't traveled as far, tastes better, and is better for the planet.

Who's in control of your food supply? Every day you can make conscious choices to eat responsibly—better for you, and better for the planet.

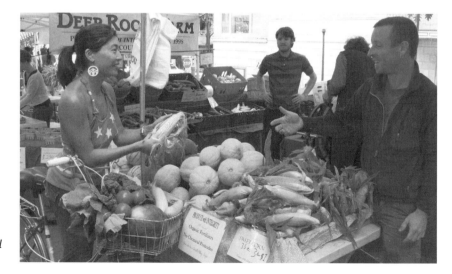

Eilif Knutson and Mark Des Marets from Deep Roots Farms hook me up with their freshest and tastiest produce at numerous farmers' markets around town several times a week.

shopping checklist

THE FOLLOWING INGREDIENTS are ones that I keep on hand in my kitchen. You won't use these all at the same rate, and you'll want to restock items as levels run low. Most of these are available at your local co-op or natural foods market. Keep in mind if you need to special order or order online, you'll be stocking your pantry for a while, so you might want to order more at one time.

FRESH HERBS AND SPICES

I prefer these herbs fresh, since the dried version sometimes tastes different. Keep the following fresh staples on hand; they'll last a couple weeks at least.

In my recipes, I've opted middle-of-the-road for garlic and chilies. Feel free to increase or decrease to your liking. I actually use double what I recommend in these recipes, but not everyone loves garlic and heat like I do. You'll notice raw garlic tastes and smells different from cooked. It doesn't make me stink as bad when it's raw. I actually think it smells good.

❏ **Ginger**
❏ **Garlic**
❏ **Onions**
❏ **Jalapeño Chilies**

Depending on my menu or mood for the week, I'll pick up the following herbs fresh. These'll only last about a week.

❏ **Basil (Italian and Thai)**
❏ **Parsley (Italian, Mexican, Spanish, Middle Eastern, Greek)**
❏ **Cilantro (Mexican, Thai, African, Indian)**
❏ **Mint (Thai, African, Middle Eastern, Indian)**
❏ **Dill (Middle Eastern, Greek)**

DRIED HERBS AND SPICES

I always keep dried spices around. They last for a really long time. I keep mine stored in labeled glass jars.

- ❏ Oregano, ½ cup
- ❏ Rosemary, ¼ cup
- ❏ Thyme, ¼ cup
- ❏ Black pepper, ¼ cup
- ❏ Curry powder, ½ cup
- ❏ Garam marsala, ¼ cup
- ❏ Turmeric, ¼ cup
- ❏ Cumin seeds, ½ cup
- ❏ Cumin, ground, ½ cup
- ❏ Cinnamon, ground, ½ cup
- ❏ Paprika or cayenne, ground, ¼ cup
- ❏ Cardamom, ground, ¼ cup
- ❏ Wasabi powder, ½ cup
- ❏ Mustard seeds, ¼ cup
- ❏ Bay leaf, 10 leaves
- ❏ Nutmeg, ¼ cup
- ❏ Psyllium powder, ¼ cup
- ❏ Poultry seasoning (a mix of sage and thyme), 1/4 cup

VANILLA BEANS OR VANILLA EXTRACT

I'm in love with vanilla beans. They can be expensive, so I buy a pound at a time to get the best deals. I use them like crazy. They really add a great dimension and flavor.

I throw the entire pod into my high-speed blender, bark and all. If you're using a less powerful blender, you might want to use alcohol-free vanilla extract instead.

Originating with the Maya, the Spaniards brought vanilla back to Spain to use as a medicine and aphrodisiac. In the 1700s vanilla was used by doctors to ensure male potency. Neurologist Alan Hirsch of the Smell and Taste Treatment and Research Foundation in Chicago has tested volunteers by having them wear masks with different scents. He found men were most aroused by the smell of vanilla. Besides being a love drug, I use vanilla beans every day, because they just taste amazing and add great flavor to mylks, smoothies, and desserts.

Vanilla beans come in several different varieties. Madagascar vanilla beans, available in the bulk section of natural food stores, are my bean of choice.

Look for fresh beans with a rich, full aroma that are oily to the touch and sleek in appearance. Beans to avoid are those with very little scent or that are smoky, brittle, or dry.

The outer "bark" on whole beans is tough, but easy to pulverize in a high-speed blender. Otherwise, you'll need to cut the beans lengthwise and scrape out the seeds inside before using. If you're feeling strained for time, you can also use an alcohol-free vanilla extract. Whenever vanilla bean is called for in the recipes, use the whole bean unless "scraped" is specified.

Vanilla beans will keep indefinitely in a cool, dark place in an airtight container. Don't refrigerate beans, as this can cause them to harden and crystallize.

- ❏ **3 vanilla beans, and/or**
- ❏ **vanilla extract, alcohol-free**

NUTS AND SEEDS

Nuts are fruits with a hard outer shell enclosing a kernel. Seeds are contained inside fruits and are capable of reproducing a new plant.

Raw nuts and seeds are a protein staple in a living-food kitchen. Most keep for many months. Some are high in oils and go rancid faster, so I store them in glass jars in the fridge or freezer.

Nuts and seeds can be expensive, so you may want to make your way down the list and choose your favorites to start, rather than buying these all at once.

If you choose only one nut, almonds have diverse uses and are an excellent nut to keep on hand. They're a great source of protein, magnesium, zinc, calcium, folic acid, and vitamin E.

Sunflower seeds provide the full spectrum of essential amino acids and are an excellent source of vitamin E, the body's primary fat-soluble antioxidant. Plus, they're the least expensive.

Make sure all nuts and seeds are untoasted, unheated, raw, and unshelled. Start with a pound of each nut or seed, unless noted otherwise.

- ❏ Almonds
- ❏ Sunflower seeds
- ❏ Flax seeds, tan or brown, keep refrigerated; or flax meal, if you don't have a way to grind whole seeds, keep frozen.
- ❏ Cashews
- ❏ Sesame seeds, tan and black – ½ lb
- ❏ Hemp seed nut – ½ lb, keep refrigerated
- ❏ Pecans
- ❏ Pumpkin seeds
- ❏ Coconut, dried and shredded
- ❏ Hazelnuts, also known as filberts, keep refrigerated
- ❏ Pistachios, ½ lb
- ❏ Brazil nuts, keep refrigerated
- ❏ Macadamias, keep refrigerated – ½ lb
- ❏ Walnuts
- ❏ Pine nuts, keep frozen – ½ lb

NUT AND SEED BUTTERS

Most nuts and seeds can be ground into a butter, like peanut butter (though raw peanut butter doesn't taste so good). Make sure to buy raw butters. If the label doesn't say raw, then it's toasted.

Different prices generally are indicative of quality when it comes to most butters, and usually the more expensive coconut butters have more coconut flavor. This ingredient is used sparingly, so it's worth it to splurge for higher quality and better flavor. Coconut butter is high in saturated fat and should be limited in your diet.

- ❏ Almond butter
- ❏ Tahini, tan and/or black
- ❏ Coconut butter, also known as coconut oil
- ❏ Cashew butter

DRIED FRUITS

Dried fruits are a great way to add healthy sweetness to a cereal or dessert. And they keep for a long while out of the fridge. Make sure to buy dried fruits that are not sulfured or sweetened with sugar.

Dried pineapple, apricot, mangoes, apples, and other fruits are good to have on hand, too, but these are my favorites and most available.

- ❏ Raisins
- ❏ Cranberries
- ❏ Goji berries

SWEETENERS

I've always had a crazy sweet tooth. What I love about live foods are the guilt-free desserts and smoothies!

Dates

My first choice for a sweetener is whole fresh dates, and they come in many varieties, each with its own unique flavor. Explore Medjool, for a maple flavor; Halawy, for a caramel flavor; and Deglet Noor, for a honey flavor. Fresh dates are actually ripened on the tree; they're not dried, as one might think.

Using dates as a natural sweetener instead of processed bleached white sugar is good for our bodies! Dates provide fiber, potassium, thiamine, riboflavin, niacin, vitamin B_6, iron, magnesium, and pantothenic acid. These vitamins and minerals help maintain a healthy body, metabolize carbohydrates, and maintain blood glucose levels and fatty acids for energy. They also help make hemoglobin, the red and white blood cells. Magnesium is essential for healthy bone development and energy metabolism.

One serving of chopped dates is equal to ¼ cup. The National Cancer Institute recommends you eat a minimum of five servings of fruits and vegetables a day for better health. This recommendation is part of a low-fat, high-fiber diet to help reduce the risk of some types of cancer.

Agave syrup is questionably raw and highly processed. All agave syrup is extracted from the agave plant by heating it between 116 and 118 degrees. There's no way to extract the syrup at only 104 degrees. The debate is over how many of the enzymes are destroyed or damaged when the temperature is raised to 118 degrees for a shorter period versus a longer period of time. Once extracted, the syrup is then processed and filtered into a clear and smooth texture. A few of my recipes will call for agave syrup as a sweetener. It doesn't contain any fiber, and it's a lot of sugar to take in all at once, even at a lower glycemic level. Used moderately, it is a good way to add sweetness without adding thickness to a texture.

Maple syrup is definitely *not* raw, but tastes really good. Go for the USDA grade B. It's usually made toward the end of the season as the weather warms into spring and the trees end their winter dormancy. Grade B is darker in color than grade A, has a stronger flavor, and contains more nutrients and minerals.

Honey is not vegan, but it's "bee"gan. Local honey is a great way to boost your immune system against allergies, since you're ingesting local pollen gathered by the bees. Make sure to use raw honey.

- ❏ **Dates, 2 pounds, keep refrigerated in airtight container**
- ❏ **Agave syrup, raw, store at room temperature**
- ❏ **Maple syrup, grade B, store at room temperature**
- ❏ **Honey, raw, store at room temperature**

SALTS

Salt can be added to your dishes in several forms. Feel free to adjust to your liking in each recipe, or to eliminate salt from any recipe.

Sea salts are high in minerals.

SEA SALT VS. IODIZED SALT

Sea salt refers to unrefined salt from a living ocean or sea. Ocean water is collected into large clay trays, where the sun and wind evaporate it naturally. Sea salt contains over seventy trace elements, enzymes, and minerals like iron, magnesium, calcium, potassium, manganese, zinc, and iodine. And they're easy for our bodies to absorb and use, because they haven't been heated. Sea salt is healthier and more flavorful that traditional table salt.

Celtic sea salt is harvested from the Atlantic seawater off the coast of Brittany, France. These salts are hand harvested using the Celtic method of wooden rakes, allowing no metal to touch the salt. Himalayan salt comes from the Himalayas and is over 250 million years old. It claims to be the purest salt available, uncontaminated with any toxins or pollutants. Sea salt also comes from the Mediterranean Sea and the North Sea.

Iodized table salt is the most common kind found in kitchens and restaurants. It comes from salt mines and is dried at over 1,200° Fahrenheit, which alters the natural chemical structure of the salt and further causes the potential for many health problems in your body. Minerals are removed from it until it's pure sodium chloride; iodine and moisture absorbents are then added to it. Iodized salt is the unnatural salt.

Miso and Nama Shoyu are both fermented and contain friendly bacteria. Unpastuerized miso has active enzymes, so it is a better choice for you than a pasteurized one. Miso paste usually comes in a tub, available at the natural food store or an Asian market.

Nama Shoyu is liquid, just like soy sauce, and should be available at most natural food stores. It is the only unpasteurized and unheated soy sauce on the market, and it's a healthy source of living enzymes and beneficial organisms like lactobacillus. It does contain wheat and gluten, which some people are allergic to.

Bragg Liquid Aminos is a gluten-free soy substitute. It's not fermented or heated, and claims to be a living food. A great substitute for those with gluten allergies, it also costs much less than Nama Shoyu. You'll want to use it sparingly, otherwise its strong flavor will dominate your creations.

I like to have both Nama Shoyu and Bragg on hand to use interchangeably. They both taste similar to soy sauce, but taste slightly different from each other.

- ❑ **Sea salt or Himalayan salt**
- ❑ **Unpasteurized miso – white**
- ❑ **Nama Shoyu**
- ❑ **Bragg's Liquid Aminos**

OILS

Oils from plant sources (vegetable and nut oils) do not contain any cholesterol. In fact, no foods from plant sources contain cholesterol.

You'll want to buy flax and hemp oils only in dark-colored bottles, as they go rancid easily and need to be kept away from light. Keep flax and hemp oils refrigerated. Once you open them, they are generally good for six months to a year or so.

- ❑ **Extra virgin cold-pressed olive oil**
- ❑ **Flax oil, keep refrigerated**
- ❑ **Hemp oil, keep refrigerated**

OLIVES

Generally, unripe olives are green and fully ripe olives are black (a few varieties are green when ripe and some turn a shade of copper brown). I always look for olives cured with sea salt, rather than conventional iodized salt. Truly raw organic olives are available from raw stores and can be mail-ordered online. My favorite place for live olives is Living Tree Community Foods in Berkeley, California (http://livingtreecommunity.com). They're cured with sea salt and never heated.

- ❑ **Black mission olives**

APPLE CIDER VINEGAR

Apple cider vinegar is the most common raw vinegar. It's high in malic acid, which helps digest proteins. And it aids construction of red blood vessels and is high in potassium. Look for raw and unfiltered.

Vinegars vary in strength. So taste yours and use it accordingly. I get a really nice raw apple cider vinegar, which is a bit lighter than others, so you may want to use a bit less. Taste first.

❑ Apple cider vinegar

SEA VEGETABLES

Raw uncooked sea vegetables offer the broadest range of minerals of any food, containing virtually all the minerals found in the ocean—which are the same minerals found in human blood. Plus, they contain lignans, plant compounds with cancer-protective properties. Sea vegetables come in many varieties that vary from sheets to strips to flakes to threads. Have fun discovering your favorite.

Nori sheets are great for making rolls and wraps, and the others are good for adding to salads and soups. Make sure your nori is labeled "raw," otherwise, it'll be toasted. Start with one package of each of the following—they're my favorites.

❑ Nori sheets
❑ Hijiki
❑ Wakame
❑ Dulse flakes

CAROB VS. COCOA, ALSO KNOWN AS CACAO

Carob is a legume that's rich in sucrose and is about 8 percent protein. It's high in vitamins A and B and several important minerals. Carob has only one-third the calories of chocolate. And where chocolate is half fat, carob is virtually fat-free. It's rich in pectin, is nonallergenic, has abundant protein, and has no oxalic acid, which interferes with absorption of calcium.

It's easier to find toasted carob powder than raw, but some co-ops will carry raw carob powder. You can also order it raw online.

Carob has been used as a caffeine-free substitute for chocolate. I actually just prefer the flavor of carob better than chocolate. If you need that caffeine kick, at least try to enjoy your chocolate raw. You'll notice the buzz is different from the toasted variety. Cocoa is also called cacao when referring to the whole beans or nibs. Cocoa and cacao come in whole beans, smaller pieces called nibs, and powder. Make sure it's raw.

Store carob and cacao/cocoa in airtight containers at room temperature.

- ❑ **2 cups raw carob powder**
- ❑ **2 cups raw cacao or cocoa powder, nibs, or beans**

FRUITS AND VEGETABLES

Lemons, limes, and some fruits last for a week or two. But greens only last a week. So buy just enough to minimize waste.

These last a couple of weeks, so I always make sure to have them on hand. These amounts are for making food for four people.

- ❑ **Lemons, 3**
- ❑ **Limes, 2**
- ❑ **Broccoli, 1 bunch**
- ❑ **Carrots, 3**
- ❑ **Celery, 1 bunch**
- ❑ **Cabbage, red, green, or Chinese, 1 head total**

The following staples generally only last a week; I always have them on hand:

- ❑ **Sprouts, 1 pint**
- ❑ **Greens, 2 to 3 heads of kale, spinach, collard, romaine**
- ❑ **Bok choy, etc.**
- ❑ **Avocado, 2 to 4**
- ❑ **Apples, 3**
- ❑ **Bananas, 4 to 6**

These lists are my staples; of course, various recipes will call for a variety of fruits and vegetables, so refer to them for more fresh fruit and vegetable ideas.

MORE SUPER FOODS

Additional super foods to keep stocked are maca root powder, spirulina, and hemp protein powder.

Maca comes from the Andes of Peru. It's a root vegetable and medicinal herb, and looks like a turnip. Maca's great for rebuilding our adrenal glands and has reported beneficial effects for sexual function due to its high concentration of proteins and vital nutrients. Look for it in powder form. My brand of choice is Maca Magic maca powder (www.macamagic .com). I keep it stored in an airtight container in the fridge.

Spirulina, a blue-green algae, is packed with chlorophyll and protein (spirulina is 65 to 71 percent *complete* protein, with all essential amino acids in perfect balance). It helps our bodies regenerate at the cellular level. There are many brands available; my favorite is VitaMineral Green from Health Force Nutritionals, a blend of spirulina and other mineral-rich foods. It comes as a powder that's easy to use and travel with. Once opened I store in the fridge, but keep it at room temperature when traveling.

Hemp protein powder is a gluten-free, vegan, and raw source for essential amino acids along with omega 3 and omega 6 essential fatty acids. Living Harvest and Manitoba Harvest are both great brands for raw hemp products. I keep all my hemp products in the fridge for immediate use, where they have about an 8- to 10-month shelf life, and store in the freezer to extend shelf life to 14 months or so.

Super foods can be found in the supplements area of your natural food store, or you can order them online.

- ❏ Maca root powder
- ❏ Spirulina
- ❏ Hemp protein powder

USING THESE RECIPES

All recipes make four servings, except the pies, cobblers, and cakes in the desserts section.

I recommend making double or triple batches so you have treats on hand in the fridge always. Mylks, dressings, pâtés, and soups keep for several days. Some desserts will keep for a week.

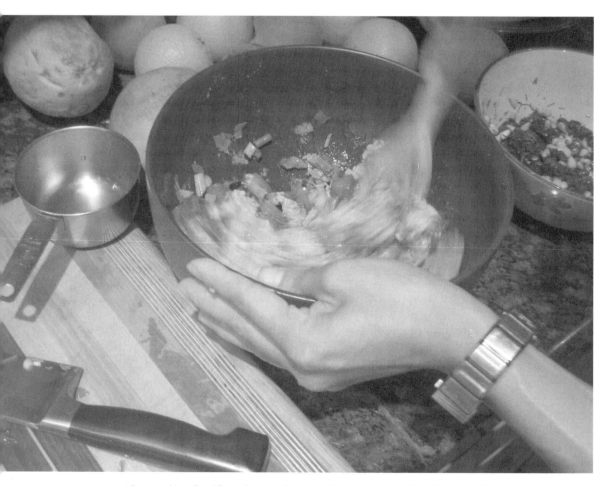

I love making food for others and inviting friends over to chow down on the dishes I create. And I make sure to ask about food allergies or dietary restrictions they may have.

You'll notice some recipes have nutritional information. It's fun to see how packed full of nutrients these foods are. Please remember when eating raw whole foods, calories and fat don't matter the same way as in cooked foods. Raw fats are good for us, and keep our organs healthy and our skin glowing. All values are estimates provided by SmartMonkey's food lab. Nutritional information is based on four servings per recipe, except where noted in the desserts section, and percent daily values are based on a 2,000 calorie diet.

Water

When recipes call for water, use filtered water if possible. I actually prefer using coconut water from a Thai baby or green coconut when it's available. It tastes amazing and provides valuable electrolytes. Coconut water is my favorite.

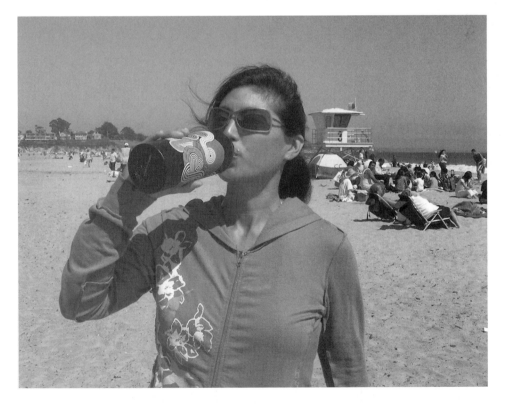

I avoid plastic water bottles that leach carcinogens into the water, especially as the plastic heats up and ages. This lightweight Sigg Swiss stainless steel bottle has been tested to prove 0 percent leaching. Plus, it keeps single-use plastic bottles out of our landfills.

Soaking nuts and seeds

It's always a good idea to soak nuts and seeds before eating. This may seem like extra work at first, but it's good for you and makes the nuts and seeds easier to digest. This mimics nature, where nuts or seeds are eaten by a bird or animal. They're then dropped into the earth, at which time their enzyme inhibitors are broken and they begin germinating. This is when the seed or nut is beginning to produce a plant, and life. It's this life force I enjoy energizing my body with.

To soak, I simply place my nuts and seeds in a glass bowl and cover with at least double the amount of filtered water before I go to bed. In the morning, I rinse them really well, *never* reusing the soak water since it contains the enzyme inhibitors. I'll place rinsed nuts in the fridge until ready to use later that day.

Sometimes my recipes call for dry nuts. So if you do soak nuts, make sure they're completely dry before using in that particular recipe. You can simply air dry by placing rinsed nuts onto a sheet tray and rotating every couple hours until dry, or place in your dehydrator for a few hours at 104° F.

Nuts are a great on-the-go energy snack. A naturally perfect balance of protein, fat, and fiber, nuts curb my hunger when I'm between kitchens.

Substitutions

DATES

Dates are my first choice for sweetener. But feel free to substitute with these other sweeteners.

AGAVE SYRUP

Substitute: ¼ cup agave syrup for ¼ cup dates.

MAPLE SYRUP

Substitute: ¼ cup maple syrup for ¼ cup dates.

HONEY

Substitute: ¼ cup honey for ¼ cup dates.

VANILLA

Substitute: 1 tablespoon vanilla extract for 1 vanilla bean.

CACAO VS. COCOA VS. CAROB

You can use cacao nibs, whole beans, or powder interchangeably. Feel free to substitute caffeine-free carob powder for cocoa one to one, and vice versa. And if you can't find cacao or carob raw at your natural food store, order it online, or use the toasted version instead.

SOY SAUCES

Feel free to use Nama Shoyu and Bragg Liquid Aminos interchangeably. Bragg has a strong unique flavor, so use it sparingly to avoid its flavor dominating your creations.

Substitute: 1 tablespoon Nama Shoyu for ½ tablespoon Bragg, adjust taste to your liking.

I hope you'll enjoy the recipes in this book so much you'll want to make them for your friends and family, too. It's a great way to introduce people to live foods. Sometimes I won't bother to tell people my dish is uncooked. All they notice is its super flavor.

I hope to encourage you to include more fresh ingredients in your daily diet. Everyone can benefit from adding a salad, or even eating an apple each day. Notice what works for you, and how good it makes you feel. Try to do better each day for yourself. It's not about extremes. You don't have to suddenly eat only live foods to experience the benefits. This is a gradual lifestyle shift that'll help you live better and feel your best.

Along the way, you'll notice that you're producing less garbage. And perhaps that your recycling bin is growing. Throughout this book, I'll talk about small things we can do to help decrease greenhouse gases, decrease garbage in our landfills, live healthy, and be happy.

I'm not at all about extremes, and I hope to inspire you to do whatever little things you can each day to improve your health along with the health of our planet.

Now let's create some taste-bud-delighting goodies!

1

drinks
for radiance

rocket fuel for my body

WHOLE, FRESH, UNPROCESSED natural foods are packed full of nutrients like vitamins, minerals, proteins, antioxidants, and enzymes. They are rich in nutrients and easy for the body to break down and use. Without fillers or chemicals, whole fresh organic food burns clean, without leaving residue behind.

QUALITY OVER QUANTITY

Organic whole foods are nutrient dense. With no fillers, you can eat less and get more nutrition in each bite.

Energy. The fresher my food, the more life energy it has. Since we're all energy, I believe it makes me vibrate at a higher frequency. For me, it's a spiritual thing.

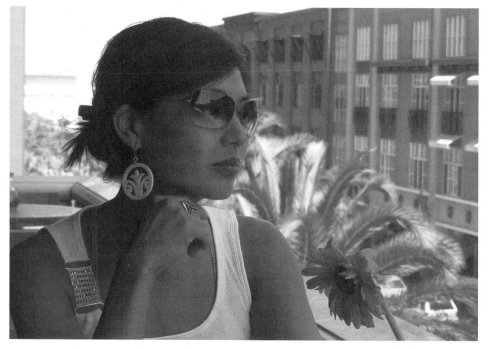

After a workout, I hydrate my body with electrolyte-rich coconut water and protein smoothies stored in glass bottles and 0 percent leaching stainless steel.

GOOD FOR THE PLANET

The freshest place to get produce is at your local farmers' market, where buying local and direct saves on transportation and packaging resources. And buying organic means no chemicals in our soil or water supply.

WHAT YOU SEE IS WHAT YOU GET

With living foods, there's no secret ingredient added to extend shelf life or alter flavor. It's all just real whole fresh goodness.

UNDERSTANDING WHERE OUR FOOD COMES FROM

I always need to know what I'm putting into my body. I figure food's the most intimate thing I buy. Unlike the clothes and shoes that dress the outside of me, food goes *into* my body and builds who I become. You are what you eat! And my body isn't a bargain body. Just 'cause a food's cheap or free doesn't mean I need to eat it.

Malnutrition is a major problem on our planet, and scientists are on a quest to feed the world. They're creating genetically engineered (GE), also known as genetically modified (GM), foods. Unfortunately, these lack proper nutrients such as vitamins, minerals, and enzymes. And we still don't know what the long-term effects of GE foods are. For example, GE foods contain antibiotic resistant marker genes used to determine if a gene has inserted itself into the plant. These crops contribute to further antibiotic resistance, which the world medical community sees as a serious public health concern.

Plus, GE crops are contaminating organic farms, because birds eat it and fly to another field, sometimes even in another country, where their droppings fertilize other soil and leach into the DNA of the non-GE crop.

At the same time, science creates preservatives to lengthen shelf life, and artificial colors to keep food looking appetizing. Striving to increase profit margins, packaged food manufacturers swap out real food ingredients for flavor and texture-altering chemicals. An emulsifier added to water, for example, creates a thickener so you don't need to use as much real juice in a drink. Using a flavoring over the fresh option means longer shelf life and lower ingredient costs. Live-food enthusiasts believe many of these chemicals and additives are the root cause of lots of illnesses, including cancer.

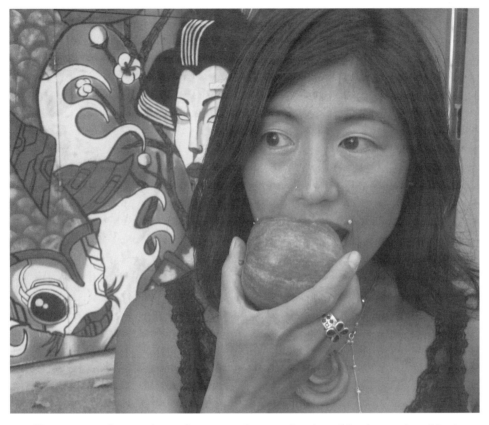

Just like no two apples are identical, variances between batches of food are a sign of fresh ingredients.

NOT LIKE THE OTHER

In nature, no two apples look identical. Our foods should also vary between batches. Think about processed and packaged cookies—they look identical cookie to cookie, because there's nothing about them that's natural or even good for our health. Variances in foods are a sign of fresh ingredients in the mix.

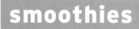

smoothies

DELICIOUS BLENDED FRUIT combinations, sometimes with nuts for added creaminess.

Use fresh fruit when it's in season, or frozen for more of a slushy texture on a hot day. When using frozen, you may need to add a little water to help keep things moving in the blender. I prefer using whole fruit to fruit juices, because whole fruit has more fiber, which makes me feel more satisfied.

For a colder drink, add in a cup of ice and blend for 5 seconds just before serving.

All smoothies will last a few days in your fridge.

VERY BLUEBERRY

MAKES 4 SERVINGS

> **3 cups water**
> **2 cups blueberries**
> **1/2 cup cashews**
> **1/2 cup pitted dates**
> **1 vanilla bean**

Blend 2 cups of water with blueberries, cashews, dates, and the vanilla bean until smooth. Add the remaining water and blend until smooth.

Will keep for three days in the fridge.

MANGO LASSI

MAKES 4 SERVINGS

> 3 cups water
> 2 mangoes, peeled, seeded, and cubed
> ¼ cup almonds
> ½ cup pitted dates
> 1 vanilla bean

Blend 2 cups of water with mangoes, almonds, dates, and the vanilla bean until smooth. Add the remaining water and blend until smooth.

Will keep for three days in the fridge.

CAROB STRAWBERRY BLISS

MAKES 4 SERVINGS

> 3 cups water
> 2 cups strawberries
> ¼ cup almonds
> ½ cup pitted dates
> ½ vanilla bean
> 1 teaspoon raw carob powder

Blend 2 cups of water with strawberries, almonds, dates, vanilla bean, and carob powder until smooth. Add the remaining water and blend until smooth.

Will keep for three days in the fridge.

PIÑA COLADA

MAKES 4 SERVINGS

3 cups water
2 cups cut pineapple
1/2 cup almonds
1/2 cup pitted dates
2 tablespoons coconut oil
1/2 vanilla bean

Blend 2 cups of water with pineapple, almonds, dates, and coconut oil until smooth. Add the remaining water and blend until smooth.

Optional: Use Thai baby coconuts, if they're available. Replace the coconut oil with coconut water and the scraped coconut meat (see *Ani's Kitchen Tip: Opening and Scraping a Young Thai Coconut* [page 139].

Will keep for three days in the fridge.

PEAR FROSTY

MAKES 4 SERVINGS

2 pears, seeded and quartered
1/2 cup pitted dates
1/2 vanilla bean
2 cups water
1 cup ice

Blend pears, dates, vanilla bean, and water until smooth. Add ice and blend 10 seconds. Serve immediately.

Will keep for three days in the fridge.

BLACK SESAME JEWEL

MAKES 4 SERVINGS

My mom tells me that in Asia black sesame seeds are so powerful they're known to restore color to gray hair. I'm still waiting for the color to come back into my grays! Regardless, sesame seeds are a great source of calcium.

2 tablespoons black sesame tahini
1 cup walnuts
½ cup pitted dates
1 vanilla bean
3 cups water
1 cup ice

Blend the tahini, walnuts, dates, vanilla bean, and water until smooth. Add the ice and blend for 5 seconds. Serve immediately.

Will keep for four days in the fridge.

PER SERVING: calories 270, protein 7g, carbohydrate 14g, fat 20g, sugar 7g
PERCENT DAILY VALUES: potassium 7%, calcium 6%, iron 7%, magnesium 15%, zinc 9%, manganese 53%, dietary fiber 13%

ANI'S KITCHEN TIP

De-seeding Vanilla Bean

BEGIN BY SLICING your vanilla bean lengthwise in half with a sharp knife. You'll see thousands of tiny seeds inside the pod.

Next, use a blunt butter knife or spoon to scrape the seeds out from the inside of the bean.

Use these seeds in your recipes.

Save your vanilla bean "bark," and put it in your jar of nuts to give them the essence of vanilla. The bark still has a ton of flavor, so use it in your high-speed blender when making smoothies.

shake it up

SO GOOD, YOU'LL want to shake your bootie!

The creaminess of blended nuts and seeds makes these shakes decadently rich and thick.

For a colder drink, add in a cup of ice and blend for 5 seconds just before serving.

BRAZILIAN CAROB SHAKE
MAKES 4 SERVINGS

> 1 cup Brazil nuts
> 1/2 cup pitted dates
> 1 vanilla bean
> 1 tablespoon raw carob powder
> 3 cups water

Blend the nuts, dates, vanilla bean, carob powder, and water until smooth.

Will keep for four days in the fridge.

VANILLA COCONUT SHAKE
MAKES 4 SERVINGS

> 1 cup pecans
> 1/2 cup pitted dates
> 1 vanilla bean
> 2 tablespoons coconut oil
> 3 cups water

Blend the pecans, dates, vanilla bean, coconut oil, and water until smooth.

OPTIONAL: Use Thai baby coconuts, if they're available. Replace the coconut oil and water with coconut water and the scraped coconut meat (see *Ani's Kitchen Tip: Opening and Scraping a Young Thai Coconut* [page 139].

Will keep for four days in the fridge.

STRAWBERRY COCONUT SHAKE

MAKES 4 SERVINGS

> **3 cups strawberries, hulled**
> **1/2 cup cashews**
> **1/2 cup pitted dates**
> **1/2 vanilla bean**
> **2 tablespoons coconut oil**
> **2 cups water**

Put strawberries in the blender, then the cashews, dates, vanilla bean, oil, and water.

Blend until smooth.

> OPTIONAL: Use Thai baby coconuts, if they're available. Replace the coconut oil and water with coconut water and the scraped coconut meat (see Ani's *Kitchen Tip: Opening and Scraping a Young Thai Coconut* [page 139].

Will keep for three days in the fridge.

CHERRY MALT

MAKES 4 SERVINGS

> **2 cups cherries, pitted**
> **3/4 cup almonds**
> **1/2 cup pitted dates**
> **2 tablespoons carob powder**
> **2 tablespoons coconut oil**
> **2 cups water**

Put cherries in the blender, then the almonds, dates, carob powder, oil, and water.

Blend until smooth.

Will keep for three days in the fridge.

PEACHY KREAM

MAKES 4 SERVINGS

1 cup peaches, pitted and diced
1 cup Brazil nuts
½ cup pitted dates
½ vanilla bean
2 cups water

Put peaches in the blender, then the nuts, dates, vanilla bean, and water. Blend until smooth.

Will keep for three days in the fridge.

FUZZY NAVEL

MAKES 4 SERVINGS

2 oranges, peeled, seeded, and sectioned
1 cup pecans
½ cup pitted dates
1 vanilla bean
1 cup water

Put oranges in the blender, then the pecans, dates, vanilla bean, and water. Blend until smooth.

Will keep for three days in the fridge.

CAROB ALMOND DECADENCE

MAKES 4 SERVINGS

> **1 cup almonds, dry**
> **1/2 cup pitted dates**
> **1/2 vanilla bean**
> **2 tablespoons carob powder**
> **2 tablespoons coconut oil**
> **3 cups water**

Put the almonds, dates, vanilla bean, carob powder, oil, and water in the blender and blend until smooth.

> OPTIONAL: Use Thai baby coconuts, if they're available. Replace the coconut oil and water with coconut water and the scraped coconut meat (see *Ani's Kitchen Tip: Opening and Scraping a Young Thai Coconut* [page 139].)

Will keep for four days in the fridge.

ALMOND NOG

MAKES 4 SERVINGS

> **1 cup almonds**
> **1/2 cup pitted dates**
> **1/2 vanilla bean**
> **1 teaspoon grated nutmeg**
> **3 cups water**

Blend the almonds, dates, vanilla bean, nutmeg, and water in the blender until smooth.

Will keep for four days in the fridge.

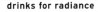

BLUE-GREEN POWER

MAKES 4 SERVINGS

I enjoy this power shake every day, and before or after a hard workout.

I use hemp and flax seeds together to balance their opposing proportions of omega 3 and omega 6 essential fatty acids. The maca is great for rebuilding the adrenal gland, which is our body's center for handling stress. It also counteracts the damage caffeine does to our adrenals. The spirulina helps my cells regenerate. The bananas provide potassium to prevent cramping.

2 tablespoons hemp protein powder
1 tablespoon maca root powder
3 tablespoons spirulina, or other blue-green algae
2 tablespoons flax seeds
2 bananas
3 cups water

Blend the hemp powder, maca root powder, spirulina, flax seeds, bananas, and water until smooth. Enjoy immediately.

PER SERVING: calories 114, protein 7g, carbohydrate 17g, fat 3g, sugar 7g
PERCENT DAILY VALUES: potassium 10%, vitamin C 9%, calcium 3%, iron 13%, vitamin E 13%, vitamin B6 17%, folate 7%, magnesium 32%, zinc 2%, manganese 18%, dietary fiber 18%

mylks

MYLKS, WHICH ARE nut and seed based, have a thin consistency, just like dairy milk for baby cows. Most of these recipes use a key secret ingredient—a pinch of sea salt. Salt adds minerals. I hear cows are given salt blocks to lick so they'll drink more water and make more milk. Which is why cow's milk has a slight saltiness to it, too.

Blend your mylk for a long time—at least 30 seconds in your high-speed blender or a minute in a conventional blender—for ultimate smoothness. Mylks will stay fresh for four to five days in your fridge.

I keep a jug of mylk in my fridge at all times to use with breakfast cereal or to simply enjoy when I'm thirsty. Sometimes I'll use it instead of water in smoothies.

VANILLA MYLK

MAKES 4 SERVINGS

This is a basic mylk that I make sure to always have in the fridge, just like the cow's milk most people keep as their staple. It tastes great as a creamer for teas and smoothies, too.

½ cup almonds
½ cup pitted dates
1 vanilla bean
Pinch sea salt
5 cups water

Put the almonds, dates, vanilla bean, salt, and water in the blender and blend until smooth.

Will keep for four days in the fridge.

COW-FREE MILK AND CREAM

Holy cow! Dairy without the milk?

I call my milks and creams "mylk" and "kream" to eliminate any confusion of it being related to animal dairy. Animal-free vegan mylk is always cholesterol free, and better for your health and our planet. And it's cruelty free.

My mylks and kreams are simply made by blending together nuts and/or seeds with water. That's faster, easier, and cleaner than going out to the barn and milking the cow.

CHOCOLATE MYLK

MAKES 4 SERVINGS

Here's the delicious chocolate version of the basic mylk recipe. I keep this on hand as a treat, for when I need a caffeine buzz, and as a way to add chocolate to my cereals.

½ cup almonds
½ cup pitted dates
3 tablespoons cocoa powder or cacao nibs
Pinch sea salt
5 cups water

Put the almonds, dates, cocoa powder, salt, and water in the blender and blend until smooth.

Will keep for four days in the fridge.

PER SERVING: calories 141, protein 5g, carbohydrate 15g, fat 8g, sugar 8g
PERCENT DAILY VALUES: potassium 7%, calcium 6%, iron 7%, vitamin E 21%, riboflavin 9%, phosphorus 10%, magnesium 17%, zinc 5%, copper 16%, manganese 23%, dietary fiber 16%

CINNAMON BANANA BUTTERMYLK

MAKES 4 SERVINGS

3 ripe bananas
2 teaspoons ground cinnamon
½ cup cashew butter
Pinch sea salt
4 cups water

Put the bananas, cinnamon, cashew butter, salt, and water in the blender and blend until smooth.

Will keep for two days in the fridge.

OPTIONAL: You can swap cashew butter for the same amount of almond butter.

YUM YUM MYLK

MAKES 4 SERVINGS

The sesame tahini used in this mylk is a great source of calcium. (Plus, black sesames are thought to have super powers, like bringing color back into your gray hairs!)

> **½ cup almond butter**
> **2 tablespoons black sesame tahini**
> **½ cup pitted dates**
> **½ vanilla bean**
> **Pinch sea salt**
> **5 cups water**

Put the almond butter, tahini, dates, vanilla bean, salt, and water in the blender and blend until smooth.

Will keep for four days in the fridge.

PER SERVING: calories 280, protein 7g, carbohydrate 19g, fat 20g, sugar 8g
PERCENT DAILY VALUES: potassium 11%, calcium 11%, vitamin E 14%, thiamin 11%, riboflavin 12%, niacin 8%, folate 8%, phosphorus 23%, magnesium 28%, zinc 9%, copper 23%, manganese 39%, dietary fiber 13%

MADE IN MEXICO MYLK

MAKES 4 SERVINGS

Inspired by my love of Mexican hot chocolate, which is rarely done up vegan.

> **¼ cup almonds**
> **½ cup pitted dates**
> **1 vanilla bean**
> **1 teaspoon ground cinnamon**
> **½ tablespoon carob powder**
> **5 cups water**

Put the almonds, dates, vanilla bean, cinnamon, carob powder, and water in the blender and blend until smooth.

Will keep for four days in the fridge.

CHOCOLATE-HAZELNUT MYLK

MAKES 4 SERVINGS

½ cup hazelnuts
2 tablespoons black sesame seeds or black sesame tahini
2 tablespoons cacao nibs
½ cup pitted dates
Pinch sea salt
5 cups water

Put the hazelnuts, sesame seeds, cacao nibs, dates, salt, and water in the blender and blend until smooth.

Will keep for four days in the fridge.

BEAUTIFYING PUMPKIN MYLK

MAKES 4 SERVINGS

Pumpkin seeds are a great source of omega essential fatty acids. Along with balancing hormone levels, essential fatty acids are known to help your skin glow.

½ cup pumpkin seeds
½ cup pitted dates
½ vanilla bean
Pinch sea salt
5 cups water

Put the pumpkin seeds, dates, vanilla bean, salt, and water in the blender and blend until smooth.

Will keep for four days in the fridge.

CASHEW BANANA MYLK

MAKES 4 SERVINGS

    2 ripe bananas
    1/2 cup pitted dates
    1/2 cup cashews
    1/2 vanilla bean
    Pinch sea salt
    5 cups water

Put the bananas, dates, cashews, vanilla bean, salt, and water in the blender and blend until smooth.

Will keep for two days in the fridge.

PRALINE MYLK

MAKES 4 SERVINGS

    1/2 cup pecans
    1/2 cup pitted dates
    1 tablespoon coconut oil
    1/2 vanilla bean
    Pinch sea salt
    5 cups water

Put the pecans, dates, oil, vanilla bean, salt, and water in the blender and blend until smooth.

Will keep for four to five days in the fridge.

juice

WITH ALL THEIR vitamins, minerals, and chlorophyll, green juices are mega-mineralizing.

When my body needs some extra minerals and vitamins, when I'm on the road and not eating as well as I'd like, or when I've got a lot on my plate and need a bit of extra TLC, I'll enjoy a green vegetable juice. Unlike fruit juice, green veggies provide minerals without so much sugar. Fruit juices, on the other hand, contain a lot of sugar that's been stripped away from fiber. A glass of orange juice is made from squeezing about five oranges. If you tried eating five whole oranges, it wouldn't be easy, because the fiber would fill you up. Nature's perfect; she packages the perfect ratio of fiber to sugar in an orange. She never intended for us to strip away the fiber to take in all that sugar at once as a juice. It's the fiber that time-releases sugar into our bloodstream.

GREEN MACHINE
MAKES 4 SERVINGS

> **2 cups spinach, washed well**
> **2 cucumbers or 4 stalks celery**
> **Any or all of the following:**
> **1 bunch parsley, washed well**
> **1 lemon, peeled**
> **1 tablespoon ginger, whole**

Juice all your ingredients in a vegetable juicer. Drink immediately.

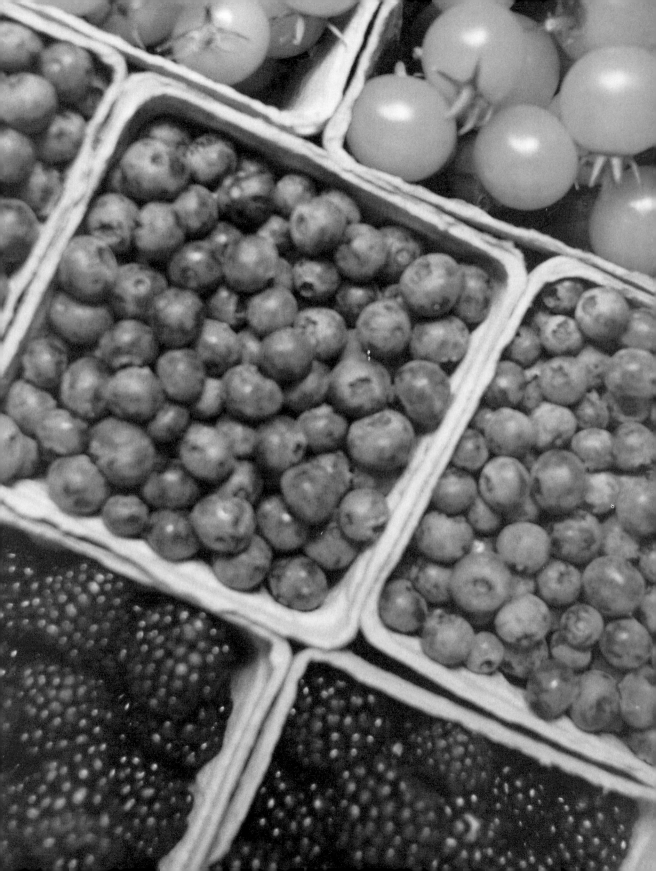

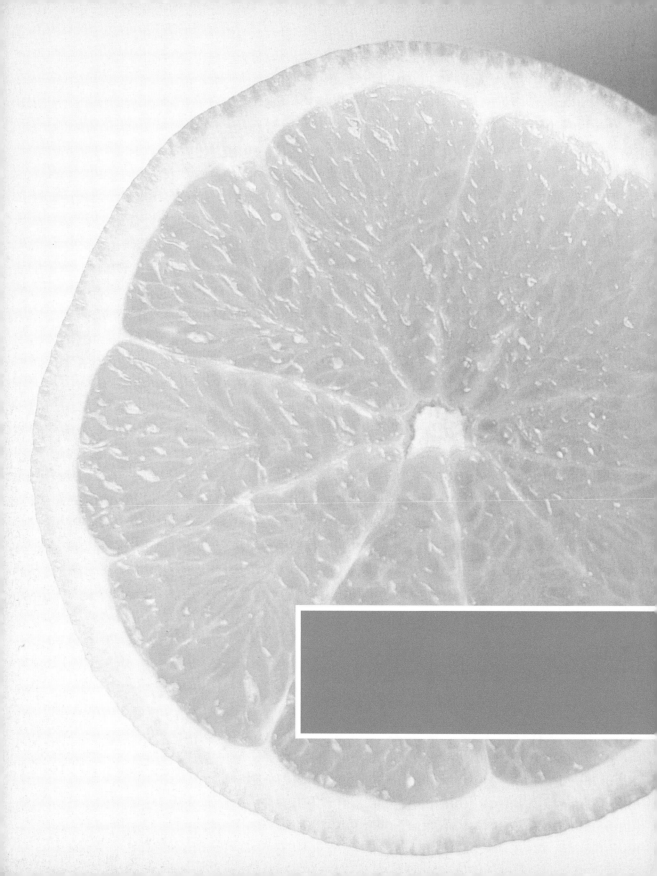

2

breakfast
of champions

green energy

NUTRIENT-RICH FOODS give you a jump start and help you get the most out of each and every day. Just like clean wind and solar energy, whole fresh organics are the cleanest fuel for my body and mind.

STAMINA

Living foods will help keep your body fine-tuned. I still surprise myself when I exercise. Last summer I went swimming in a river. It had been years since I'd been swimming, but when I came out, I was shocked to discover I'd been swimming for fifty minutes! It's the same with running. Even if I don't run for a year, I can go out and run five miles as if I'd just run yesterday.

ENDURANCE

I love my sleep. But there are times when sleep just isn't a priority. I've had to decrease my sleep to just a couple hours a night. And amazingly, I never get sick. Before I understood the benefits of a living-foods diet, I'd get sick several times a year. I'd get the stuffed-up nose and fever illness that was just miserable. Now, rather than being forced to take downtime because I'm sick, I'm free to choose to take my downtime in the form of a break or holiday.

MENTAL CLARITY

You'll notice an increase in your mental clarity through living foods. Energy that would otherwise be spent digesting food is directed to your brain to help it think more clearly, and helps it orchestrate the trillions of cells in your body.

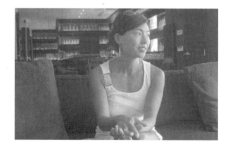

FOCUS

The brain's a muscle and needs fuel in the form of nutrients to hum. Living foods are packed full of all the right nutrients like vitamins, minerals, and oxygen to feed the brain all it needs to run at its best.

PRODUCTIVITY

My increase in mental clarity, focus, and endurance has had quite an impact on my productivity. New friends are surprised to hear about all the projects I'm working on at any given time, and how quickly and efficiently I complete them all. Friends who've known me awhile just expect me to be hyperactive. Some call me the energizer bunny!

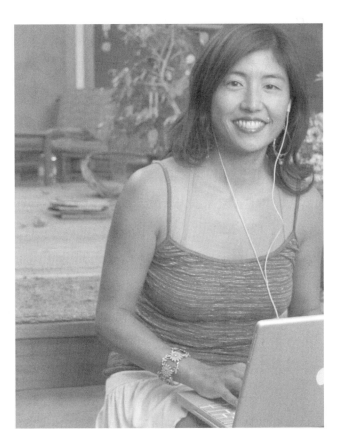

cereals

THESE CEREALS ARE made with nuts, seeds, fruit, and my Buckwheat Crispies (you'll find the recipe below). They are a delicious fresh alternative to the standard processed breakfast cereals that are full of preservatives.

Enjoy these cereals with your favorite mylk.

BUCKWHEAT CRISPIES
MAKES 4 CUPS

I like to make a couple pounds of Buckwheat Crispies at a time, and then store them in an airtight jar. They're the raw version of Rice Krispies, travel easily, and keep for at least six to nine months. Like Rice Krispies, they don't have much flavor, so you'll want to enjoy them with a delicious mylk for breakfast. And they're great for adding crunch to salads, desserts, and wraps.

Enjoy Buckwheat Crispies with your favorite mylk. Adding Chocolate Mylk (page 55) reminds me of Cocoa Krispies cereal.

1 pound buckwheat groats

Put buckwheat groats in a large bowl and fill to the top with water. The buckwheat will more than double in size as it expands, so use enough water to keep it fully under water.

I like to rinse the buckwheat every few hours to keep the water fresh. You'll notice the soak water get thick and slimy quickly. It's also fine to just leave it in the same water for the six to eight hours of soak time, too. And feel free to add water if it looks like it could use more.

Rinse soaked buckwheat thoroughly after soaking six to eight hours. If you're using an Excalibur dehydrator, put the mesh screens onto each tray. If using a dehydrator with holes larger than the buckwheat groats, you'll want to place parchment paper as a base onto each tray first. Spread buckwheat onto your dehydrator trays.

Dehydrate at 104º F for three to five hours, or until completely dry.

Sun Drying and Dehydrating

DEHYDRATORS ARE ELECTRICAL sunshine simulators used to sun dry without the sun. They come in different shapes and sizes, and are basically a box with a heating element and a fan that blows hot air around inside. Dehydrators heat up at low temperatures, unlike an oven. You may want to look for one with a timer so you don't have to be around to turn it off.

When I'm in the desert or on a hot summer day, I'll use sunshine to sun dry rather than using electricity to dehydrate. The food absorbs all the goodness of the sun, plus I'm saving energy.

I'll just take my buckwheat, spread it out on baking trays, and lay it in the sun to dry, rotating the buckwheat groats every hour or so. Depending on how hot and humid it is out, it will take about three to five hours for your Buckwheat Crispies to dry.

GOJI BERRY SUNSHINE CEREAL

MAKES 4 SERVINGS

Goji berries are considered to be one of the most nutritious food sources on the planet. They're rich in antioxidants, vitamin A, and zeaxanthin. They contain B-complex vitamins, and 500 times more vitamin C than oranges. They're 10% protein, and supply nineteen different amino acids, including all eight essential amino acids. In addition, goji berries are loaded with many phytonutrients and are used in Asia in Chinese medicine and for antiaging benefits. You can find these delectable treats at your local health food store or online.

> 1 cup goji berries
> 1 orange, peeled, seeded, and diced
> 2 bananas, sliced
> 1/2 cup figs, fresh or dried, chopped
> 1/2 cup Buckwheat Crispies (page 66)

Put the goji berries, orange, bananas, figs, and Crispies in a bowl and enjoy with mylk immediately, so your bananas won't brown.

GOOD MORNING MUESLI

MAKES 4 SERVINGS

> 2 apples or 2 peaches, diced
> ½ cup cranberries
> 1 cup pumpkin seeds
> ¼ cup black or tan sesame seeds
> ¼ cup flax seeds

Put the apples, cranberries, pumpkin, sesame, and flax seeds in a bowl and enjoy with mylk immediately.

NIRVANA HEMP MUESLI

MAKES 4 SERVINGS

Hemp seed nut is the earth's most nutritious seed. It's 33% protein, rich in vitamin E and iron, as well as omega 3, omega 6, omega 9, and GLA, and is enzyme-inhibitor-free.

Hemp is a weed, grows easily anywhere, and has no natural pests. It's grown without pesticides or herbicides, making it a safer product for our bodies and the earth. Growing hemp restores our soils and conserves forests. (Plus, it has a wonderful, delicious nutty flavor!)

> 3 bananas, sliced
> 1 cup figs, fresh or dried, chopped
> 1 cup hemp seeds
> ½ cup sunflower seeds
> ½ cup Buckwheat Crispies (page 66)

Put the bananas, figs, hemp and sunflower seeds, and Crispies in a bowl and enjoy with mylk immediately.

PER SERVING: calories 305, protein 14g, carbohydrate 35g, fat 17g, sugar 18g
PERCENT DAILY VALUES: potassium 31%, vitamin C 15%, calcium 17%, iron 21%, vitamin E 61%, thiamin 50%, riboflavin 13%, folate 20%, pantothenic acid 20%, vitamin K 11%, phosphorus 50%, magnesium 75%, zinc 22%, copper 63%, manganese 81%, selenium 978%, dietary fiber 55%

ALMOND CINNAMON OATMEAL

MAKES 4 SERVINGS

This oatmeal tastes better than the cooked version, and is so fast and easy to make. Be sure to use raw oat groats, since rolled oats and steel-cut oats are cooked while processed.

> **2 cups oat groats, soaked overnight, and rinsed well**
> **½ cup semi-soft pitted dates**
> **1 tablespoon ground cinnamon**
> **2 tablespoons water, as desired**
> **¼ cup almonds, chopped**

Put soaked oats, dates, cinnamon, and water in the food processor and process into a creamy texture similar to cooked oatmeal. For a thinner texture, add another ¼ cup of water and process.

To serve, scoop into four bowls and top each with chopped almonds.

Will keep for two days in the fridge.

OPTIONAL: Drizzle 1 teaspoon maple syrup on top of each bowl of oatmeal. I like my oatmeal really thick with a side of nut mylk.

BANANA RAISIN OATMEAL

MAKES 4 SERVINGS

> **2 cups oat groats, soaked overnight, and rinsed well**
> **3 bananas, chopped**
> **2 tablespoons water, as desired**
> **1 cup raisins**

Put soaked oats, bananas, and water in the food processor and process until mixed well. For a thinner consistency, add another ¼ cup of water and process. Add raisins last and pulse to mix them in.

Enjoy as is, or serve really thick with a side of nut mylk.

Will keep for one day in the fridge.

OPTIONAL: Drizzle 1 teaspoon maple syrup on top of each bowl of oatmeal.

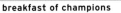

SMARTMONKEY BARS

Try cutting up a couple bars of your favorite flavor SmartMonkey Bar and use it to top any morning cereal. Or try one of these Smart-Monkey Bar recipes. Explore the flavors and delight your senses and taste buds.

SMARTMONKEY BAR OATMEAL

MAKES 4 SERVINGS

    2 cups oat groats, soaked overnight, and rinsed well
    ½ cup pitted dates
    2 tablespoons water, as desired
    2 SmartMonkey Bars, any flavor, chopped

Put oats, dates, and water in the food processor and process into a creamy texture, like that of cooked oatmeal.

Dish into four bowls and serve topped with chopped SmartMonkey Bars. Enjoy!

Will keep for two days in the fridge.

SMARTMONKEY BAR CEREAL

MAKES 4 SERVINGS

    2 apples, diced
    1 cup Buckwheat Crispies (page 66)
    1 cup sunflower seeds
    2 SmartMonkey Bars, any flavor, chopped

Put the apples, Crispies, seeds, and SmartMonkey Bars in four serving bowls. Mix well. Serve with your favorite nut mylk and enjoy immediately.

puddings

THESE PUDDINGS MAKE for a fast breakfast or a simply delicious snack. Just place ingredients into a blender or processor and voila, you've got pudding in the mix!

Try layering puddings into a parfait glass, or scoop some atop a crepe with fresh fruit for a beautiful presentation of delicious goodness. Make sure to try the parfait and crepe recipes at the end of this section.

ANI'S KITCHEN TIP

I RECOMMEND ALL nuts and seeds be soaked for at least eight hours in filtered water, and rinsed very well with fresh water before using. No need to dry them for these pudding recipes since we'll be adding more water when blending them.

CAROB PUDDING

MAKES 4 SERVINGS

2 avocados
2 bananas
¼ cup carob powder

Put the avocados, bananas, and carob powder in the food processor and process until smooth. Enjoy immediately.

CACAO PUDDING

MAKES 4 SERVINGS

2 cups almonds
1 cup water
¼ cup pitted dates
1 tablespoon cacao nibs or powder
1 tablespoon carob powder

Blend the almonds and water in the blender until smooth. Add the dates, cacao, and carob. Blend until smooth.

Will keep for three to four days in the fridge.

CASHEW COCONUT PUDDING

MAKES 4 SERVINGS

2 cups cashews
1 ½ cups water
¼ cup pitted dates
½ cup shredded dried coconut or fresh coconut

Blend the cashews and water until smooth. Add the dates and coconut. Blend until smooth.

Will keep for three to four days in the fridge.

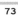

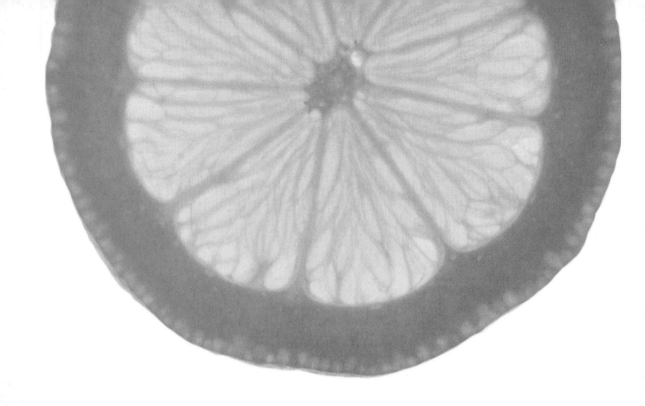

LUSCIOUS LEMON PUDDING

MAKES 4 SERVINGS

This recipe uses psyllium powder as a natural thickener. It has a unique flavor, so use it sparingly. Psyllium helps maintain healthy cholesterol and blood lipid levels. In 1998, the U.S. Food and Drug Administration authorized the health claim that diets low in saturated fat and cholesterol that include soluble fiber from psyllium may reduce the risk of heart disease by lowering cholesterol.

> **2 cups almonds**
> **1/2 cup pitted dates**
> **Juice of 1 lemon, about 2 tablespoons**
> **2 cups water**
> **2 tablespoons psyllium powder**

Blend the almonds, dates, lemon juice, and water until smooth. Add psyllium and blend well.

Will keep for three to four days in the fridge.

FRUIT PARFAIT

This is a really pretty dish, as you'll see the layers through the glass. And you'll enjoy all the flavors and textures together at once.

> **2 peaches or bananas, sliced, or 2 cups berries**
> **1 cup Buckwheat Crispies (page 66)**
> **1 recipe of your favorite pudding (pages 73–74)**

In a parfait glass, layer fruit, Crispies, and then pudding. Repeat. Enjoy immediately.

CREPE KREAM STACK

MAKES 4 SERVINGS

> **½ recipe Coconut Breakfast Cake (page 78)**
> **½ recipe of your favorite pudding (pages 73–74)**
> **1 cup fresh fruit, sliced**

Divide the Coconut Breakfast Cake batter into four balls. Flatten each ball into a thin crepe that's about ⅛ to ¼-inch thick and place onto a dish.

Serve topped with a layer of pudding and fresh fruit.

Pudding and Coconut Breakfast Cake will keep for three days in the fridge. Top with fresh fruit before eating.

inspired by pancakes

ONE OF THE main breakfast treats I missed for years was pancakes. So I was inspired to create this recipe, and I love it more than the pancakes I remember!

COCONUT BREAKFAST CAKES

MAKES 4 SERVINGS

Flax seeds are a great source of omega 3, similar to that found in fish such as salmon. Many studies have shown flax seeds lower total cholesterol and LDL cholesterol (the bad cholesterol) levels. Flax seed may also help lower blood triglyceride and blood pressure and reduce the chance of a heart attack. Flax seed is rich in fiber and the antioxidant lignan, known to fight disease and prevent cancer, especially breast cancer.

Flax goes rancid quickly, so it's ideal to keep whole seeds in your fridge and to grind just before using. But for convenience, flax seeds can be found already ground in a meal at most stores. Keep meal stored in a dark, cold place, like your freezer.

This is one of the instances where I use agave syrup for its thin watery texture. Plus, it's being added to ultra-fiber-rich flax. This fiber helps to slowly time-release sugar into our bloodstream.

These breakfast cakes are a great vehicle for your favorite syrup!

2 cups whole flax seeds, or 3 cups flax seed meal
2 tablespoons liquid coconut oil
½ cup agave or maple syrup
½ teaspoon sea salt
¼ cup water

Put flax meal, coconut oil, agave, salt, and water in a large bowl and mix well. Form four balls and flatten into a "pancake" shape, about ¼ to ½ inch thick.

To serve, top with sliced fruit like bananas and/or chopped nuts like walnuts or almonds. Drizzle with one of the syrups and a pat of "butter" (recipes follow).

Batter will keep for four to five days in the fridge.

OPTIONAL: Mix blueberries or walnuts into your breakfast cake batter.

SYRUPS

You can use maple syrup, agave, or honey on top of your Coconut Breakfast Cakes. Or for a truly raw vegan treat, try one of the following syrup recipes. They're fast and simple to make.

BERRY-LICIOUS SYRUP

MAKES 4 SERVINGS

⅓ cup pitted dates
1 pint blueberries, blackberries, or strawberries

Blend the dates and berries until smooth. Add water if needed to mix well.

Will keep for two days in the fridge.

ORANGE VANILLA SYRUP

MAKES 4 SERVINGS

⅓ cup pitted dates
1 orange, peeled, seeded, segmented
½ vanilla bean

Blend the dates, orange, and vanilla bean until smooth. Add water if needed to mix well.

Will keep for two days in the fridge.

VANILLA SYRUP

MAKES 4 SERVINGS

½ cup pitted dates, or figs, fresh or dried
¾ to 1 cup water, as needed
½ vanilla bean

Blend the dates, water, and vanilla bean until smooth. Use as much water as needed for desired consistency.

Will keep for three to four days in the fridge.

BUTTERS

Pancakes aren't complete without a slab of butter on top. Here are two fun butter recipes to drool over.

OLIVE BUTTER

This butter will come out similar to a stick of dairy butter, where you'll be able to cut off a pat in a solid shape. This recipe needs to be made ahead of time to allow for at least 4 hours of freeze time.

¼ cup extra virgin olive oil
¼ teaspoon sea salt

In a small bowl, mix oil and salt. Pour into a small container and freeze until solid. Use just like you'd use a dairy butter.

Will keep for several months in the freezer.

COCONUT BUTTER

MAKES 4 SERVINGS

This butter has a soft whipped butter texture. Start with a solid, rather than liquid, coconut oil. Miso is used to add flavor and saltiness. Use an unpasteurized miso for its living enzymes. This butter can be served as soon as you're done mixing it up.

¼ cup coconut oil
1 tablespoon white miso

Mix coconut oil and miso with a spoon or fork until mixed well.

Will keep for a couple months in the freezer.

chicken-friendly scrambles

YOU'LL ENJOY THESE guilt-free and cruelty-free scrambles. Add your favorite ingredients to the basic Love-the-Chicks Pâté for an egg-free morning delight.

LOVE-THE-CHICKS PÂTÉ

MAKES 4 SERVINGS

> 2 cups almonds, dry
> 1 cup sunflower seeds, dry
> ½ teaspoon sea salt
> 2 teaspoons turmeric
> 1 cup water

Put almonds, sunflower seeds, salt, and turmeric in a food processor and process into a powder. Add water and process until mixed well. It will have small chunks, rather than being completely creamy smooth. Use the recipes that follow, or add your favorite ingredients like mushrooms, tomatoes, and onions to this pâté base to make different "scrambles."

PER SERVING: calories 386, protein 22g, carbohydrate 11g, fat 24g, sugar 3g
PERCENT DAILY VALUES: potassium 22%, calcium 21%, iron 31%, vitamin E 176%, thiamin 65%, riboflavin 36%, niacin 21%, vitamin B6 18%, folate 25%, pantothenic acid 27%, phosphorus 57%, magnesium 77%, zinc 27%, copper 68%, manganese 119%, selenium 33%, dietary fiber 46%

GARDEN SCRAMBLE

MAKES 4 SERVINGS

1 cup red, orange, and/or green bell pepper, diced
1 cup tomato, diced
¼ cup yellow onion, diced
1 batch Love-the-Chicks Pâté (page 81)
1 cup spinach leaves or other softer greens like red leaf lettuce or butter lettuce

Place the pepper, tomato, and onion in a bowl with a batch of Love-the-Chicks Pâté. Mix well.

To serve, scoop your Garden Scramble onto a bed of spinach leaves.

Will keep for two days in the fridge.

SPANISH SCRAMBLE

MAKES 4 SERVINGS

½ cup fresh cilantro leaves
1 cup tomato, diced
¼ cup chopped scallions
1 batch Love-the-Chicks Pâté (page 81)
1 cup spinach leaves or other soft greens, like red leaf lettuce or butter lettuce
Pinch ground black pepper

Place cilantro, tomato, scallions, and a batch of Love-the-Chicks Pâté in a bowl and mix well.

To serve, scoop your Spanish Scramble onto a bed of spinach leaves. Top with black pepper.

Will keep for two days in the fridge.

ASIAN SCRAMBLE

MAKES 4 SERVINGS

> **2 cups shiitake mushrooms**
> **¼ cup Nama Shoyu or 3 tablespoons Bragg Liquid Aminos**
> **3 tablespoons extra virgin olive oil**
> **2 tablespoons black or tan sesame seeds**
> **¼ cup chopped scallions**
> **1 batch Love-the-Chicks Pâté (page 81)**
> **8 baby bok choy leaves**

Wipe mushrooms clean with a damp cloth, then slice.

Mix mushrooms, Nama Shoyu, and oil. Set aside to allow the mushrooms to marinate. After five minutes, use your hands to squeeze the excess liquid from your marinated mushrooms.

Mix marinated mushrooms, sesame seeds, scallions, and a batch of Love-the-Chicks Pâté in a large bowl.

To serve, scoop Asian Scramble onto a bed of two baby bok choy leaves per serving.

Will keep for two days in the fridge.

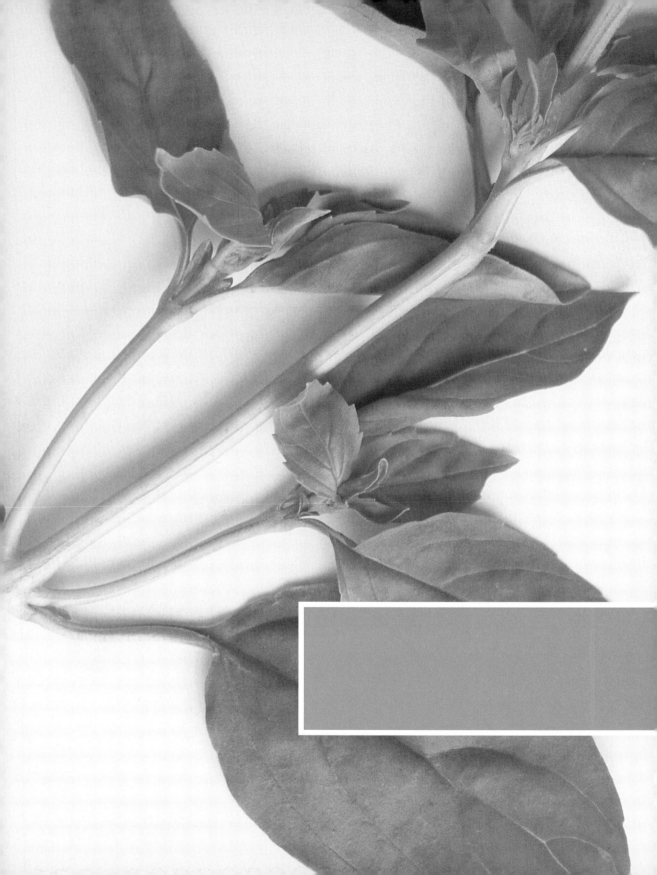

3

fresh salads
and simple dressings

a green planet

FRESH ORGANICS ARE not only healthy for us, but they also give back to the planet, because at the end of a large meal, you'll have only created a few cups of organic compost—which in turn, creates organic soil to grow more organic produce.

On the other hand, overprocessed, genetically modified, hormone-filled, and chemically toxic foods can leave a path of destruction behind. Packaged in boxes, containers, and plastics (which use lots of energy to create in the first place), it all ends up in a landfill at the end of the day.

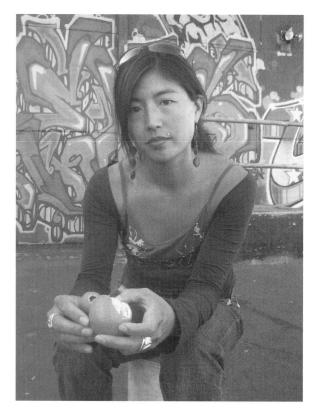

When I was living in Los Angeles, I'd trade my organic compost for produce at the local farmers' market. If this isn't an option for you, even if you end up throwing away your compost rather than trading it, the banana skin or carrot pieces will biodegrade superfast—unlike a Styrofoam cup, which takes an eternity to decompose.

The highest concentrations of carbon monoxide (CO) are found near roadways from vehicle exhaust, and cause headaches, fatigue, respiratory problems, and death. According to the EPA (from the 2002 *World*

Enjoying more delicious and nutritious fresh, whole, organic foods means you're doing good for your body while also contributing to the future of our planet. What we eat has the largest impact on the planet. We can choose to leave a path of life or a path of destruction behind with every bite.

Almanac), 97,441 thousand tons of carbon monoxide were released in the United States during 1999, about 76 percent caused by transportation exhaust. When I was living in LA, it killed me to see fourteen-lane highways and all the cars on the roads. Half of the population of Los Angeles is in their cars twenty-four hours a day. That's over six million people driving!

Here in the greener Pacific Northwest, I'm stoked to see many bio-diesel vehicles. Better yet, there's a ton of bicycles on the road, buses and trains are full of commuters, and many people everywhere are traveling on foot.

COMPOSTING

In nature, composting is what happens as leaves pile up on the forest floor and decay. Eventually, the rotting leaves go back to the soil, and living roots finish the recycling process by reclaiming nutrients from the decomposed leaves. Composting at home is the way to reduce the volume of garbage sent to landfills by recycling our yard and kitchen waste.

By composting plant remains, you can create an earthy, dark, crumbly substance that's great for adding to houseplants or enriching garden soil. If you have a yard, composting can be as simple as making a pile of organic remains and allowing them to decompose. Some folks dig a hole and rotate the compost within it daily to aide the breakdown process. If you don't have a yard, you can get a home composting bin or a worm box online for less than $100.

GARBAGE-FREE

As soon as I began eating all fresh living foods, I noticed a huge decrease in my weekly garbage. It was clear to see most of my garbage had been packaging from processed foods. Now I rarely create garbage. Rather, I create organic compost and things that can be recycled.

REUSE AND RECYCLING

You can help our planet by choosing products with less packaging, since chances are good you're going to throw that packaging away anyway. I reuse all my grocery bags and food containers until they fall apart. Then I'll recycle them. It's much better to recycle and buy products made from recycled goods than to throw things into a landfill or buy new.

While recycling is a great thing, keep in mind that the process of recycling still uses energy and creates pollution. Plus, it's important to buy items made with recycled and 100 percent post-consumer-recycled materials, made from used materials, because fewer resources and less energy were used when creating the product and its packaging. And less ends up in a landfill along the way.

I save and reuse all my jars and containers. Here I'm reusing a glass jar to store my cashew kream. Glass jars work great as glasses or cups, and they're great for storing dried herbs and spices. Plastic bags from the bulk section work just as well as a new zip lock baggie for carrying snacks with you on the go. I even use plastic bags to cover leftovers in the fridge, instead of using plastic wrap. Paper grocery bags work as well as a new garbage can for gathering recyclables like paper, plastic, and glass. The blank parts of junk mail work great for writing notes. Return mail envelopes included in solicitations or bills can be addressed and used to mail letters and other bills. Old T-shirts can be cut into fabric squares and work better than a paper towel to dust and clean around the house.

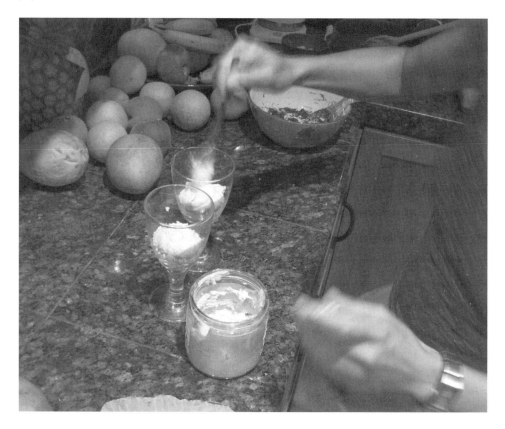

BUY IN BULK

Cut out excess packaging by buying in bulk and using your own containers. When shopping at the co-op, I'll take my own glass jars to fill with bulk items like Nama Shoyu or agave syrup. Some stores will even give you a discount for using your own containers and shopping bags. Consider buying your favorite herbs or spices a pound at a time. They'll come sealed in a vacuum-packed bag for optimal freshness. Most stores offer discounts for this, too. And most stores are happy to special-order items they might not carry regularly, such as raw carob, for example. Ordering in bulk will save you money as well.

GREEN TIP

Shop Locally for More Than Just Food

IT'S EASIER TO know where and how products were made.

Larger corporations can be greater environmental offenders. They can ravage the earth of its resources on a much larger scale and at a faster rate, and get away with it, because they can afford to pay high lawyer fees to help get them out of trouble and are able to give financial backing to politicians. And buying from a national or international chain means pollution, as products are shipped by land, air, and sea. Plus, chances are, you'll need to drive your car to visit these large chains, further adding to pollution.

Supporting your local mom-and-pop businesses keeps your money within your community. Plus, you're able to create a relationship with local businesses. This is super important, because as new cookie-cutter suburban sprawl development pushes farther out into the countryside, property values in the older parts of the community usually fall. This outward expansion of new development makes it harder to recycle while forcing people to drive everywhere, creating the need for more and more parking lots to be built over our green landscape.

Sprawl destroys community centers where people come together face-to-face frequently enough to know and trust each other. It forces us to drive in different directions to buy groceries, clothes, and stamps, lowering the chances for us to run into old friends or meet new people along our journey.

For more information, check out the National Trust for Historic Preservation's 1999 report for the Henry M. Jackson Foundation, "Challenging Sprawl: Organizational Responses to a National Problem."

SHOP AT FARMERS' MARKETS AND BUY LOCAL WHEN POSSIBLE

Buying direct from local farmers means you're getting seasonal produce that's at its peak in flavor and nutrition. And it'll be super fresh, probably picked just a few hours earlier. You'll be able to taste the difference. Besides keeping money within your local community, your food wouldn't have had to travel far.

GREEN TIP

Reuse and Recycling Fashion

REUSED CLOTHING IS as cool as reused containers and paper.

I love trading in clothes I haven't worn for a while for used clothes that are new to me. When buying new, I try to buy hemp, organic cotton, bamboo, and recycled fibers and fabrics. I like supporting local businesses promoting individual style. Creative handmade artisan garments and accessories are far more interesting to me than something everyone else is wearing.

With the shortage of cool fabrics with great prints, it's fun to turn T-shirts into fitted stylie clothes. Even without a sewing machine, you can use scissors to cut strips of fabric and use them to weave together pieces of recycled fabric. If you do know how to sew, it's fun to add details to old boring clothes using recycled fabrics. Sew fabric to the front or down the sleeve of a shirt, for example.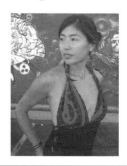

OUR GARBAGE STAYS AROUND
LONGER THAN WE THINK

More important than recycling is reducing waste of all kinds. Just by consuming less, we can make a difference. Think twice before drinking drinks that come in plastic bottles, and even buying that extra pair of shoes or pants.

A few garbage timelines:

Banana peel	3 weeks
Paper bag	1 month
Cotton T-shirt	5 months
Wool sock	1 year
Lumber	15 years
Leather shoe	50 years
Aluminum can	200–500 years
Disposable diaper	500–600 years
Plastic jug	1 million years
Glass bottle	unknown
Styrofoam	eternity

salads

THE KEY TO salads is a variety in texture and colors. You'll notice I like mixing tougher kales with softer arugula or spinach, for example. A great addition is cabbage. It comes in red, green, and Chinese varieties, and adds color and a sweet, fresh crispness. Plus, cabbage is an alkalizing vegetable. The more alkaline our bodies are, the better we're able to absorb minerals and other nutrients, increase energy production in our cells, increase our body's ability to repair damaged cells, and increase its ability to detoxify heavy metals. It also makes it harder for tumor cells to thrive, while helping combat fatigue and illness.

Most marinated and dressed salads will keep for a day, maybe two days for tougher greens like kales, in the fridge. I'd recommend storing untossed salad and dressing separately to keep each fresh longer.

A tip for eating healthy is to always have easy-to-grab options around. I like to wash and prep my greens and salad vegetables all at one time. Then I keep them in a container in the fridge so I have salad mix ready to eat always. I keep a jar of dressing on hand, too. When I'm starving, it's super convenient to grab a handful of salad mix and toss with dressing for a quick, easy, healthy snack.

SHAVED FENNEL WITH BLOOD ORANGES, POPPY SEEDS, AND MICRO GREENS

MAKES 4 SERVINGS

Micro greens are the new gourmet sprout. They're beautifully colored and incredibly tasty. As the plant's first true leaves, micro greens are harvested when they're about ½ to 2 inches high and are at their peak in nutrition and flavor.

> 1 large fennel bulb, trimmed
> 2 medium oranges, peeled
> 2 tablespoons extra virgin olive oil
> 1 teaspoon poppy seeds
> 2 cups micro greens

Shave the fennel bulb into thin slices with a knife or mandoline. Cut oranges into slices, cutting across the segments, and remove seeds.

Place oranges and fennel in a bowl and drizzle with olive oil. Let salad marinate for five to ten minutes to allow the flavors to blend.

Top with poppy seeds and micro greens and serve at room temperature.

Tossed salad will keep for one day in the fridge.

CABBAGE KALE SLAW
IN SIMPLE GREEK DRESSING

MAKES 4 SERVINGS

SALAD

½ head kale, any type, destemmed
¼ head red cabbage

SIMPLE GREEK DRESSING

2 tablespoons apple cider vinegar
¼ cup extra virgin olive oil
½ teaspoon sea salt
1 teaspoon thyme

Thinly slice the kale and cabbage with a knife or mandoline. Place kale and cabbage in large mixing bowl.

Place the vinegar, oil, salt, thyme, kale, and cabbage in the salad bowl and toss well.

To serve, enjoy immediately or set aside for ten minutes to allow slaw to soften and marinate.

Tossed salad will keep for one day in the fridge. Salad mix will keep for two days, and dressing will keep for five days when stored separately.

CONFETTI SALAD
IN ORANGE-CUCUMBER DRESSING

MAKES 4 SERVINGS

SALAD

½ head of red leaf or romaine lettuce, torn into bite-size pieces

½ bunch dinosaur kale (also known as Lacinato kale), ribs removed and leaves torn into bite-size pieces

2 cups red cabbage, chopped

1 cup walnuts

½ cup cherries, dried or fresh

ORANGE-CUCUMBER DRESSING

1 small cucumber, about 5 inches long, diced

1 medium orange, peeled, seeded, and diced

¼ cup extra virgin olive oil

¼ cup cashews

1 tablespoon grated ginger

1 clove garlic

Juice of 1 lemon, about 2 tablespoons

1 teaspoon sea salt

Place lettuce, kale, cabbage, and walnuts in a large salad bowl.

To make the dressing, place all dressing ingredients in a blender and blend until smooth.

To serve, toss salad with Orange-Cucumber Dressing. Top with cherries for color.

Tossed salad will keep for one day in the fridge. Salad mix will keep for two days, and dressing will keep for three to four days when stored separately.

ANI'S KITCHEN TIP

De-veining Garlic

I RECOMMEND DEVEINING garlic if you have the time. This means cutting the clove in half and removing any green root that has begun to sprout in the center. Removing this sprout will give you a milder flavor and make the garlic easier to digest. Most folks who have trouble digesting garlic are actually having trouble digesting the vein, and find deveined garlic fine on their system.

SPRING HERB RAINBOW IN KREAMY CURRY DRESSING

MAKES 4 SERVINGS

SALAD

½ bunch rainbow chard, tough ribs removed, leaves torn into bite-size pieces

¼ head red cabbage, cored and thinly sliced

1 bunch fresh dill, chopped

¼ bunch fresh rosemary, chopped

1 bunch fresh cilantro leaves, chopped

CREAMY CURRY DRESSING

1 tablespoon curry powder

1 apple, cored and diced

1 clove garlic

1 tablespoon grated ginger

1 cup extra virgin olive oil

Juice of 1 lemon, about 2 tablespoons

½ teaspoon sea salt

For salad, combine chard, cabbage, dill, rosemary, and cilantro in a large bowl.

To make the dressing, place all dressing ingredients in a blender and blend until smooth.

To serve, toss salad with Creamy Curry Dressing.

Tossed salad will keep for one day in the fridge. Salad mix will keep for two days, and dressing will keep for three to four days when stored separately.

EVERGREEN SALAD
IN SUNFLOWER THYME MARINADE

MAKES 4 SERVINGS

SALAD

1 bunch red kale, ribs removed, and leaves torn into bite-size pieces

1/2 bunch mustard greens, ribs removed, and leaves torn into bite-size pieces

1/2 bunch spinach, torn into bite-size pieces

1 bunch arugula, torn into bite-size pieces

SUNFLOWER THYME MARINADE

2 tablespoons fresh thyme leaves

1 clove garlic

1 cup extra virgin olive oil

1/2 cup sunflower seeds

1 tablespoon apple cider vinegar

1 teaspoon sea salt

For salad, put kale, mustard greens, spinach, and arugula in a large salad bowl. Chop leftover stems and add to salad.

To make the marinade, blend all marinade ingredients until smooth.

To serve, toss salad with marinade and let it sit at room temperature for 10 minutes before serving. The longer the greens marinate, the softer they become.

Tossed salad will keep for one day. Salad mix will keep for two days, and marinade will keep for three to four days when stored separately.

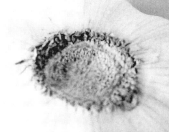

ASIAN GREENS SALAD
WITH **SUPER ASIAN DRESSING**

MAKES 4 SERVINGS

I promise any extra time you may spend finding Asian greens for this salad will be made up by the time saved making the super-easy dressing. The flavors are worth it. Many times you can even find a mix of Asian greens at the natural food store.

This salad calls for three Asian greens: mizuna, tat soi, and bok choy. Mizuna is a Japanese mild mustard with dark green, beautifully fringed leaves. Tat soi has small, green leaves with white stems that form a tight rosette. And bok choy has thick and tender white stalks and deep green leaves.

If you can't find Asian greens, substitute spinach and green cabbage.

SALAD

1 cup bok choy, thinly sliced

2 cups mizuna, torn

2 cups tat soi, torn

2 bunches watercress, bottom 2 inches discarded, cut into 1-inch pieces

1 cup basil leaves, cut into ½-inch-wide strips

1 cup cherry tomatoes

SUPER ASIAN DRESSING

1 avocado, seeded and cubed

2 tablespoons hemp oil

2 teaspoons Nama Shoyu or Bragg Liquid Aminos

1 tablespoon ginger, chopped fine

2 tablespoons tan or black sesame seeds

2 tablespoons scallions, chopped

For salad, combine bok choy, mizuna, tat soi, watercress, basil, and tomatoes in a large bowl.

For dressing, add the avocado, oil, Nama Soyu, ginger, sesame seeds, and scallions to the salad. Toss well, serve immediately.

Salad mix will keep for one day, and dressing will keep for two days in the fridge when stored separately.

THAI SALAD MIX
WITH KAFFIR LIME LEAF DRESSING

MAKES 4 SERVINGS

Fresh mint, basil, and kaffir lime leaves give this salad a burst of Southeast Asian flavor.

Kaffir lime leaves have a distinct flavor and a perfume unlike any other. Fresh leaves can be found at most natural food stores or Thai markets. If fresh kaffir lime leaves are not available, you can use the tender new leaves of lime, lemon, or grapefruit, but they won't have the same fragrance.

You may be able to find a kaffir lime tree at a plant nursery, where it will flourish even in temperate climates. So you could grow your own if you fall in love with the flavor.

SALAD

4 cups spinach, torn into bite-size pieces
¼ head Chinese cabbage, cored and sliced
1 bunch mint leaves, torn
½ bunch basil leaves, torn
2 cups mung bean sprouts

KAFFIR LIME LEAF DRESSING

1 cup extra virgin olive oil
6 kaffir lime leaves
Juice of ½ lemon, about 1 tablespoon
1 tablespoon Nama Shoyu
2 stalks celery
1 tablespoon grated ginger

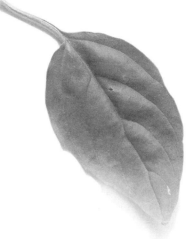

For salad, combine spinach, Chinese cabbage, mint leaves, basil leaves, and mung bean sprouts in a large salad bowl.

To make the dressing, place all the dressing ingredients in a blender. Blend until smooth.

To serve, pour dressing over salad. Toss well and serve immediately

Salad mix will keep for one day, and dressing will keep for three days in the fridge when stored separately.

WILTED SPINACH SALAD WITH MARINATED ONIONS IN MUSTARD SEED DRESSING

MAKES 4 SERVINGS

MARINATED ONIONS

½ yellow onion, sliced
1 tablespoon apple cider vinegar
1 tablespoon Bragg Liquid Aminos or Nama Shoyu
Pinch black pepper

MUSTARD SEED DRESSING

1 tablespoon soft dates or 1 tablespoon agave syrup, maple syrup, or honey
3 tablespoons apple cider vinegar
¼ cup extra virgin olive oil
1 teaspoon mustard seeds
½ teaspoon sea salt

SALAD

8 cups of spinach
2 carrots, julienned
Pinch ground black pepper

To marinate onions, combine onions with vinegar, Bragg Liquid Aminos, and black pepper. Set aside to marinate while you prepare the rest of the salad.

To make the dressing, if you're using dates, soak them in 2 tablespoons of water for 5 minutes, or until soft. Mash together the dates and water until it becomes a thick syrupy paste. Pour syrup, vinegar, oil, mustard seeds, and salt in small bowl and mix well.

For salad, place spinach and julienned carrots in a large bowl. Pour in Marinated Onions, including the marinade. Toss with Mustard Seed Dressing.

To serve, top tossed salad with a pinch or two of black pepper. Set aside for five minutes or more to allow time for wilting. Or if you're like me and can't wait, it's okay to eat right away.

Salad mix will keep for one day, dressing will keep for three to four days, and Marinated Onions will keep for one day in the fridge when each are stored separately.

ARUGULA WITH GOLDEN BEETS AND WALNUTS IN ORANGE MISO DRESSING

MAKES 4 SERVINGS

SALAD

1 bulb fennel, trimmed and quartered lengthwise

2 cups golden beets, peeled and julienned

2 scallions, thinly sliced

1 bunch arugula, torn into bite-size pieces

½ cup walnuts

ORANGE MISO DRESSING

2 tablespoons miso, preferably white

1 orange, peeled and seeded

⅓ cup extra virgin olive oil

1 tablespoon grated ginger

1 clove garlic

For salad, slice fennel with knife or mandoline. Place fennel, beets, scallions, arugula, and walnuts into a large bowl.

To make the dressing, place all dressing ingredients in a blender. Blend until smooth.

To serve, toss salad with dressing.

Tossed salad will keep for one day. Salad mix will keep for one day, and dressing will keep for three to four days in the fridge when stored separately.

SPINACH SALAD
WITH PERSIMMONS AND SPICED PECANS
IN SHALLOT LEMON DRESSING

MAKES 4 SERVINGS

There are two types of persimmons. This recipe calls for the Fuyu variety, which looks like a slightly flattened tomato. It's crisp, lightly sweet, and crunchy.

Choose Fuyu persimmons that are a rich orange color and firm to the touch. Fuyus will stay firm for a week or two at room temperature. After about two weeks, they'll soften to the texture of a firm papaya and be at their peak of sweetness. This is the time I enjoy them most.

Persimmon season is late fall into early winter. They give us betacarotene, vitamin C, and potassium—and make a beautiful holiday garnish.

SALAD
12 cups spinach leaves, torn into bite-size pieces
3 Fuyu persimmons, sliced thinly into little discs
1 batch Sweet Spiced Pecans (page 145)

SHALLOT LEMON DRESSING
1 tablespoon finely chopped shallots
Juice of 1/2 lemon, about 1 tablespoon
2 tablespoons apple cider vinegar
1/2 cup extra virgin olive oil
3/4 teaspoon sea salt
Pinch ground black pepper

For salad, place spinach and persimmon discs in a large bowl.

To make the dressing, combine shallots, lemon juice, and vinegar in a small bowl. Slowly whisk in olive oil in a small stream until well blended. Season with salt and pepper.

To serve, toss salad with dressing. Top with Sweet Spiced Pecans and serve immediately.

Salad mix will keep for one day, and dressing will keep for four days in the fridge. Sweet Spiced Pecans will keep for a week.

WAKAME HEMP POWER SLAW

MAKES 4 SERVINGS

Wakame is a delicious sea vegetable that's high in calcium and protein. It's a great source of chlorophyll, too.

SLAW

½ head of green or red kale, ribs removed, and leaves torn into bite-size pieces

¼ head red cabbage, cored and thinly sliced

2 scallions, chopped

½ cup dry wakame

½ cup hemp nuts

POWER DRESSING

¾ cup Brazil nuts

2 cloves garlic

1 tablespoon grated ginger

1 teaspoon sea salt

¼ cup hemp oil

Juice of 1 lime, about 2 tablespoons

¼ cup water

For slaw, cut or tear kale leaves from stem, and thinly slice leaves. Place in a large bowl with sliced cabbage, scallions, and wakame.

To make dressing, process nuts, garlic, ginger, and salt until mixed well. Add oil, lime, and water, and process until smooth. Scoop into bowl with slaw. Toss well.

To serve, top with hemp nuts.

Tossed slaw will keep for one day. Slaw mix will keep for two days, and dressing will keep for four days in the fridge when stored separately.

PER SERVING: calories 430, protein 8g, carbohydrate 11g, fat 22g, sugar 2g
PERCENT DAILY VALUES: potassium 13%, vitamin A 56%, vitamin C 50%, calcium 12%, iron 11%, vitamin E 26%, thiamin 21%, riboflavin 5%, vitamin B6 7%, folate 10%, vitamin K 197%, phosphorus 35%, magnesium 47%, zinc 14%, copper 43%, manganese 61%, selenium 1200%, dietary fiber 17%

PERFORMANCE POWERHOUSE POST-WORKOUT FUEL

Wakame Hemp Power Slaw is a great pre- and post-workout food. Besides tasting really good, the hemp nuts and Brazil nuts are a great source of protein. Ginger acts as an anti-inflammatory, which is great after a hard workout. Plus the entire slaw is packed full of chlorophyll for even more protein plus calcium.

VIRTUES OF SEA VEGETABLES AND DARK GREENS

Sea vegetables are one of nature's richest sources of complete vegetable protein (up to 38%) and vitamin B12. Ounce for ounce, sea vegetables are higher in essential vitamins and minerals than any other food group, and are a great source of potassium, calcium, magnesium, iron, iodine, chlorophyll, enzymes, and fiber. Sea vegetables vary in shape, color, and texture. Nori comes in sheets used for sushi rolls, wakame and hijiki come in strands, and dulse comes in strands or flakes, to name a few.

Sea vegetables have a balancing, alkalizing effect on the blood. They are known for their ability to reduce cholesterol, remove metallic and radioactive elements from the body, and to prevent goiter.

Thought to have cancer-fighting benefits, sea vegetables also provide relief from asthma, thyroid disorders, irritable bowel syndrome, and reduce cholesterol and blood pressure.

Everything that's green has chlorophyll to thank. And the darker the green, the better. Chlorophyll's chemical structure is similar to that of our red blood cells. The only difference is that the center of our red blood cell is iron, while the center of chlorophyll is magnesium. This makes it really easy for our body to assimilate chlorophyll nutrients. Plus, chlorophyll is one of the highest sources of protein on the planet. Ounce for ounce, it provides more than any animal product.

BLACK SESAME ASIAN SLAW
WITH GINGER CASHEW MAYO

MAKES 4 SERVINGS

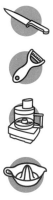

SLAW

4 cups Chinese cabbage
1 carrot, julienned
1 cup mung bean sprouts
2 scallions, chopped
¼ cup black sesame seeds

GINGER CASHEW MAYO

2 tablespoons ginger
1 clove garlic
1 teaspoon sea salt
2 cups cashews
Juice of 1 lemon, about 2 tablespoons
¼ cup water, as needed

SLAW TOPPINGS

¼ cup dry hijiki
¼ cup cilantro leaves, lightly chopped

For slaw, slice cabbage with knife or mandoline slicer. Place in a large bowl with carrot and sprouts.

For Ginger Cashew Mayo, process ginger, garlic, and salt in a food processor until finely chopped. Then add cashews and process into powder. Add lemon juice and process, adding water as needed to make a creamy "mayonnaise." Toss with salad. Then add the scallions and sesame seeds and toss lightly.

For slaw toppings, soak dry hijiki in about ¼ cup filtered water, just enough to barely cover it. Set aside to rehydrate and soften for a few minutes.

To serve, place salad onto four serving bowls. Squeeze excess water from soaked hijiki, and use to top each slaw. Garnish with cilantro, and serve.

Tossed slaw will keep for one day. Slaw mix will keep for two days, dressing will keep for four days, and slaw toppings will keep for two days in the fridge when each are stored separately.

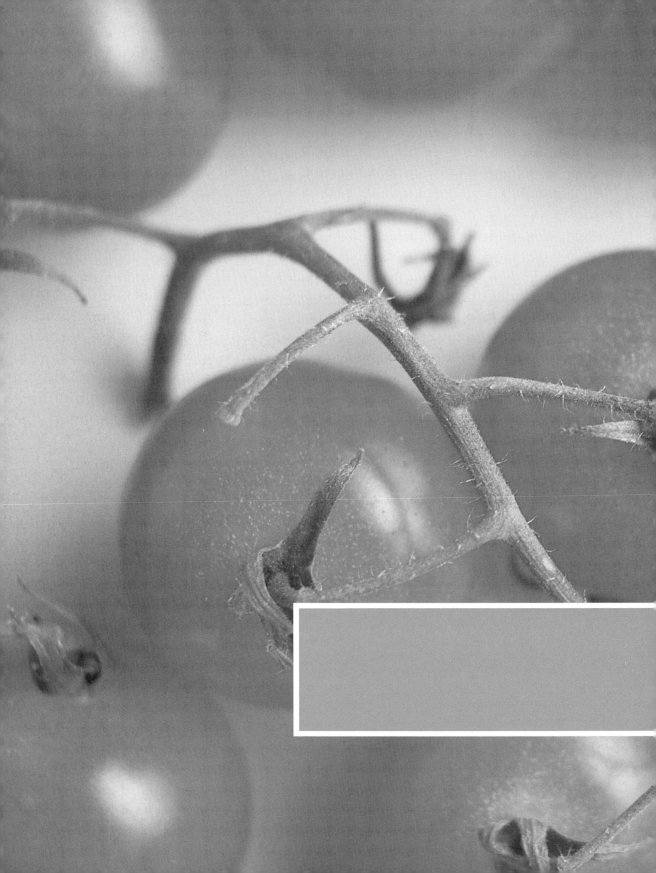

4

soups and sauces to tickle your tongue

the joy of uncooking

UNCOOKING IS AN art form for me. It's all about the textures and flavors and simulating cooked versions of dishes we crave. My living-food recipes are inspired by their cooked recipes. I take note of the herbs, spices, and special flavors. If I've eaten the dish before, I remember the texture and think creatively about how to mimic it. Thinly sliced zucchini may replace cooked pasta. Or Buckwheat Crispies (page 66) may replace Rice Krispies. Even carrot pulp is great as the fiber for mock fish salads and fish cakes.

Raw-living soups aren't too much different from their cooked versions, except they're not served piping hot. It's possible to heat up your soups in your blender by keeping it running on high. But you want to watch it to make sure it doesn't heat up too much. Just stick your finger in it, and stop when it's slightly warm to your touch. In colder months, I like to add heat in the form of spicy hot chili peppers, ginger, and garlic.

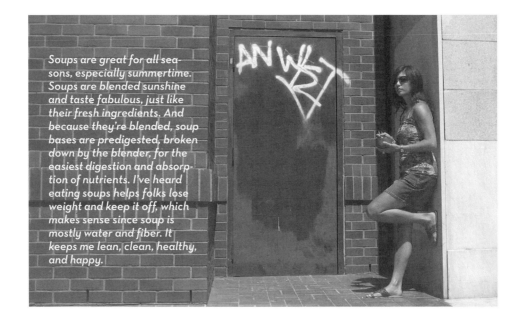

Soups are great for all seasons, especially summertime. Soups are blended sunshine and taste fabulous, just like their fresh ingredients. And because they're blended, soup bases are predigested, broken down by the blender, for the easiest digestion and absorption of nutrients. I've heard eating soups helps folks lose weight and keep it off, which makes sense since soup is mostly water and fiber. It keeps me lean, clean, healthy, and happy.

FRESHNESS

Uncooking is about freshness. Starting with the freshest ingredients, uncooking preserves the water content, fiber, nutrients, enzymes, and flavor. Even the color stays vibrant. Think about the wan color of overcooked broccoli—not very appetizing!

GREEN TIP

Preserve Biodiversity, Eat Heirlooms

HEIRLOOM PRODUCE is high in nutrients and rich in aroma, color, and taste. We are what we eat. If we choose fresh, organic, locally grown crops, we are supporting gardeners and farmers who choose to maintain our right to good food. Avoiding the environmental impact of international shipping, the exploitation of migrant and developing-nation workers, as well as unnecessary chemical exposure makes heirlooms and the preservation of our biodiversity important.

There are hundreds of heirloom crops to explore, including cucumbers, lettuces, radishes, squashes, peppers, eggplants, melons, and of course tomatoes.

UNCOOKING SAVES RESOURCES

I don't use a stove to cook. This means I'm not buying, using, or disposing of a big metal stove. That's one less large appliance in a landfill that takes thousands of years to decompose, if at all.

Choosing not to use a stove means no carbon monoxide is being released into my environment or into the atmosphere. Across the country, more than ten million Americans use woodstoves, and a single dirty woodstove emits as much fine-particle pollution as seven old dirty diesel buses.

When using a gas stove, make sure it's adjusted properly to decrease the amount of emissions, ventilate and increase the amount of outdoor air coming inside by opening windows and doors, and consider using an air cleaner or filter. For more information, visit www.EPA.gov.

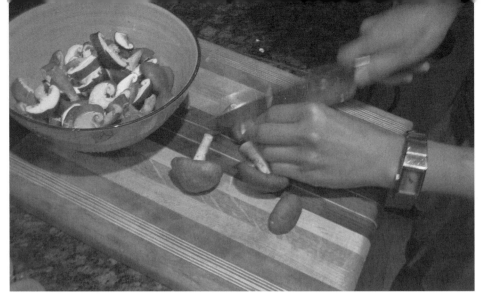

It's easy to marinate mushrooms with olive oil and Nama Shoyu or Braggs. In just a few minutes, they'll soften and feel "cooked," without fire or electricity.

GREEN TIP

Pedal Power Your Appliances

ALL THE CARS on the roads and the burning of fossil fuels are affecting human health and our atmosphere. Better known as global warming, it's changing our climate.

Pedal power, energy created by riding a bike, means less pollution. And it conserves energy. It uses the most powerful muscles in our body to covert 95 percent of exertion into energy.

A table saw, water pump, stone polisher, pottery wheel, and many appliances like juicers, blenders, coffee grinders, grain mills, TVs, and washing machines can all run on pedal power. You can exercise, save energy, and make a smoothie all at once!

There are also hand-crank appliances like ice cream makers, blenders, flashlights, and radios. These are great for camping and traveling. It's nice to know I can still make food by candlelight in a blackout.

For more information, check out the Fender Blender, a pedal-powered stationary bike fitted with a blender. And visit sites like www.alternative-energy-news.info/pedal-power/ for do-it-yourself plans to build a pedal generator.

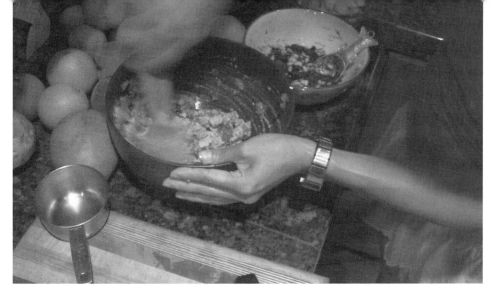

Easy to make—and easy to clean!

EASY CLEANUP

The thing I really like about raw foods is the easy cleanup. No more cooked or baked-on crust to soak and scrub, scrub, scrub. Instead, all it takes is water to rinse and sometimes a wipe with a sponge and some Dr. Bronner's Soap.

When I'm making several dishes, I'll rinse out my blender between each savory recipe and just wash once before moving on to a sweet recipe.

NO CONTAMINATION

Since I'm not dealing with animal products, there's no worry of cross-contamination of bacteria like E. coli, and I don't have to worry about disinfecting surfaces and sponges all the time. Even the USDA health department is more lenient in our commercial kitchen than in other cooked kitchens. There just aren't as many cleanliness issues with fresh live foods. Fresh, organic, vegan, whole foods not only clean our bodies, but they *are* also clean.

VEGAN

I understand that some people enjoy meat and that a vegan diet is not for everyone. Animal products work for some, but I choose to keep my home vegan. This means no animal products are allowed inside at all. This frees me up from having to worry about keeping things sterile and disinfected all the time.

MEAT OR NOT?

It wasn't a huge, dramatic conversion. One night when I was in college, my friends and I hit a late-night drive-thru for burgers. One bite, and I decided it wasn't for me. The taste and texture just weren't appetizing to me. So I made a decision at that point not to eat meat anymore. Over the years, I've experienced better health and have become more in tune with my love for animals.

I LOVE ANIMALS

Along my journey to vegetarian, vegan, and now living foods, my connection to animals has deepened. I feel more compassion for all living beings.

Modern factory farming crowds animals into such unhealthy conditions, they need antibiotics to survive. The animals are given hormones to make them grow bigger and faster than nature intended. Simply put: these chemicals enter our environment and our bodies and stick around for a long while.

MY PATH TO VIBRANT HEALTH

When I began eating a lot of dairy products in college, my cholesterol became dangerously high. Rather than taking the pharmaceuticals my doctor recommended, I cut out all animal products like my raw-food-enthusiast mother suggested. My bad cholesterol levels dropped in a flash.

Along with my high cholesterol, I suddenly became allergic to pets, even though I'd grown up with several dogs and had never had any problems. I also noticed seasonal allergies to pollen. Within a month of becoming 100 percent raw, all my allergies disappeared.

According to the Vegetarian Society's food allergy and intolerance information sheet, symptoms from food intolerances include asthma, eczema, hives, fatigue, and migraines, to name a few. Not all food intolerances are related to meat and dairy products, but vegetarians and vegans suffer less from food intolerance because they already eliminate most of the common causes of intolerance, which include milk, eggs, fish/shellfish, wheat/flour, artificial colors, pork, chicken, cheese, and yeast.

LEAVE NO TRACE, TREAD LIGHTLY ON OUR PLANET

The biggest burden our diet places on our planet is from meat and animal products. Livestock eat a large percentage of our grain crops, require millions of gallons of water, and give off waste that pollutes rivers, groundwater, and soil.

The earth's livestock population is more then three and a half times its human population. Raising livestock takes up more than two-thirds of our agricultural land, and one-third of the total land area.

We just don't have enough land to feed everyone on an animal-based diet.

Eight hundred and forty million people don't have enough food to live normal lives. But we continue to waste two-thirds of our agricultural land to raise livestock when we could be growing food to feed the world instead.

FEED PEOPLE RATHER THAN COWS

Over 60 percent of U.S. grain is fed to livestock. Livestock are increasingly being fed grains and cereals that could instead be directly eaten by humans, or were grown on land that could be used to grow human food rather than animal feed.

The developing world's undernourished millions are competing with the developed world's livestock for food. And the humans are losing.

EARTH-FRIENDLY VEGAN SHOES, ACCESSORIES, AND MORE

Even Stella McCartney, daughter of vegetarians Paul and Linda McCartney, offers beautifully designed non-leather shoes and bags. Vegan shoes made from human-made materials are eco-friendly, usually cheaper than leather, and longer wearing. Car upholstery, coats and jackets, furniture, wallets, purses, and handbags are all available in leather alternatives such as fabric, fake fur, recycled PET (plastic drink) bottles, microfiber, canvas, and vinyl. MooShoes.com is one of the many online vegan accessory and clothing stores.

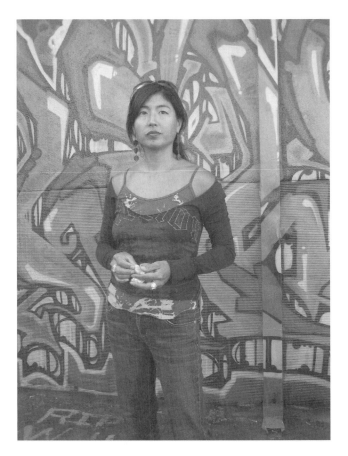

There's more vegan fashion available today than ever before.

nourishing soups

TEXTURE AND PRESENTATION are key in live-food preparation. That's why you'll notice most of my soups are made up of two parts: the smooth soup base and the chunky toppings for texture and visual color.

Stir your soup base before serving if it sits for a while. And make sure to add soup toppings last, just before serving.

You might want to make double or triple batches of your recipes. It's easy to keep soup base in the fridge, then add toppings before serving. Soup bases keep up to four or five days in your fridge,. Store base and toppings separately to preserve freshness.

HEIRLOOM TOMATO GAZPACHO

MAKES 4 SERVINGS

SOUP BASE

3 tomatoes, heirloom if possible
1 tablespoon pitted dates
1/2 cup Brazil nuts
1 cup extra virgin olive oil
2 cloves garlic
1 teaspoon ground black pepper
1 tablespoon Nama Shoyu or Bragg Liquid Aminos
4 cups water

SOUP TOPPINGS

1 large tomato, heirloom if possible, diced
1/2 cucumber, peeled and diced
1/2 bunch of cilantro leaves

Blend tomatoes, dates, Brazil nuts, oil, garlic, pepper, Nama Shoyu, and water until smooth.

To serve, pour soup base into four soup bowls. Add diced tomato and cucumber toppings to each soup bowl. Top with cilantro leaves and serve.

Soup base with toppings will keep for one day. Soup base will keep for three days, and toppings will keep for one day in the fridge when stored separately.

ANI'S KITCHEN TIP

GARLIC WALNUT SOUP

MAKES 4 SERVINGS

SOUP BASE

1 cup walnuts

1 cup extra virgin olive oil

2 cloves garlic

½ teaspoon ground black pepper

1 teaspoon sea salt

2 ½ cups water

SOUP TOPPINGS

2 avocados, diced

¼ bunch fresh dill, chopped

Blend walnuts, oil, garlic, pepper, salt, and water until smooth.

To serve, pour soup base into four soup bowls. Top each with avocado and fresh dill.

Soup base with toppings will keep for one day. Soup base will keep for four to five days, and toppings will keep for one day in the fridge when stored separately.

CREAMY PORTABELLO BISQUE

MAKES 4 SERVINGS

BISQUE BASE

1 cup Brazil nuts

1 cup extra virgin olive oil

2 cloves garlic

1 teaspoon sea salt

3 cups water

BISQUE TOPPINGS

1 portabello mushroom, diced

¼ cup extra virgin olive oil

1 tablespoon Nama Shoyu or Bragg Liquid Aminos

1 tablespoon fresh thyme leaves

Start by marinating your mushroom pieces. Toss them with oil and Nama Shoyu. Set aside to marinate.

Blend nuts, oil, garlic, salt, and water until smooth.

To serve, pour bisque into four soup bowls. Top each with marinated portabello and thyme.

Soup base with toppings will keep for two days. Soup base will keep for four to five days, and toppings will keep for two days in the fridge when stored separately.

JAPANESE MISO-SHIITAKE SOUP

MAKES 4 SERVINGS

SOUP BASE

3 tablespoons miso, white or brown

1 cup extra virgin olive oil

1 tablespoon grated ginger

1 clove garlic

3 cups water

SOUP TOPPINGS

3 cups shiitake or oyster mushrooms, sliced

2 tablespoons Nama Shoyu or Bragg Liquid Aminos

3 tablespoons extra virgin olive oil

1 scallion, chopped

Start by marinating your mushrooms. Toss shiitake mushrooms with Nama Shoyu and oil. Set aside to marinate.

Blend miso, oil, ginger, garlic, and water until smooth.

To serve, pour soup base into four bowls. Top each with marinated mushrooms and scallions.

Soup base with toppings will keep for one day. Soup base will keep for four days, and toppings will keep for two days in the fridge when stored separately.

TOMATO BASIL BISQUE

MAKES 4 SERVINGS

BISQUE BASE
3 tomatoes, chopped

2 cloves garlic

1 ½ cups extra virgin olive oil

2 teaspoons sea salt

2 cups water

BISQUE TOPPINGS
1 tomato, diced

1 cup basil chiffonade (see below)

Blend three tomatoes, garlic, oil, salt, and water until smooth.

To serve, pour bisque base into four bowls. Top each with tomatoes and basil.

Soup base with toppings will keep for one day. Soup base will keep for two days, and toppings will keep for one day in the fridge when stored separately.

ANI'S KITCHEN TIP

Chiffonade Your Basil

Chiffonade means cutting into long, thin strips. First, stack five to ten basil leaves on top of one another. Next, roll the leaves into a tight cylinder, lengthwise. Slice the cylinder widthwise into very thin strips.
There you have it! Basil chiffonade.

LEMON FENNEL SOUP

MAKES 4 SERVINGS

This is a light and refreshing brothlike soup base with sliced fennel and scallion.

For lunch on the lighter side, serve with a salad. Or try serving it with a creamy pasta, such as Pad Thai Noodles in Almond Kaffir Sauce (page 186) or Fettuccini Squash Noodles in Alfredo Sauce (page 182).

SOUP BASE

Juice of 2 lemons, about 1/4 cup

3 cups water

1/2 cup extra virgin olive oil

1 1/2 teaspoons sea salt

1 clove garlic, minced

SOUP TOPPINGS

1/2 fennel bulb, about 1/2 pound, thinly sliced

1 scallion, sliced

Whisk lemon juice, water, oil, salt, and garlic in a large bowl.

To serve, pour soup base into four bowls. Top each soup with fennel and scallion.

Soup base with toppings will keep for one day. Soup base will keep for three days, and toppings will keep for two days in the fridge when stored separately.

PER SERVING: calories 250, protein 1g, carbohydrate 3g, fat 19g, sugar less than 1g
PERCENT DAILY VALUES: potassium 4%, vitamin A 2%, vitamin C 19%, calcium 2%, iron 3%, vitamin E 17%, vitamin K 22%, phosphorus 2%, magnesium 2%, manganese 4%, dietary fiber 4%

SWEET CORN CHOWDER

MAKES 4 SERVINGS

CHOWDER BASE

3 ears sweet corn
¾ cup walnuts
¾ cup extra virgin olive oil
1 clove garlic
1 teaspoon sea salt
2 cups water

CHOWDER TOPPINGS

1 cup corn kernels, set aside from above
1 avocado, diced
⅓ bunch cilantro leaves
1 teaspoon cracked black pepper

Set aside 1 cup of corn kernels to use as chowder topping.

Blend remaining corn, walnuts, oil, garlic, salt, and water until smooth.

To serve, pour chowder base into four bowls. Top each with corn, avocado, cilantro, and a pinch of cracked black pepper.

Chowder base with toppings will keep for one day. Chowder base will keep for two days, and toppings will keep for one day in the fridge when stored separately.

THAILAND TOM KHA GAI

MAKES 4 SERVINGS

SOUP BASE

4 celery stalks, chopped

2 cloves garlic

4 kaffir lime leaves

3 tablespoons coconut oil

1 cup extra virgin olive oil

1 to 2 teaspoons Thai cayenne

1 ½ teaspoons sea salt

4 cups water

SOUP TOPPINGS

1 head baby bok choy or 1 leaf regular bok choy, sliced

1 ½ cups broccoli florets, broken into small pieces

1 cup cherry tomatoes, halved

2 avocados, cubed

½ bunch cilantro leaves

Blend celery, garlic, lime leaves, coconut oil, olive oil, cayenne, salt, and water until smooth.

To serve, place sliced bok choy in bottom of four soup bowls. Pour soup base into bowls. Top with remaining soup toppings.

Soup base with toppings will keep for one day. Soup base will keep for four days, and toppings will keep for one day in the fridge when stored separately.

SPICY KREAM OF AVOCADO SOUP

MAKES 4 SERVINGS

SOUP BASE

3 avocados

¼ cup miso, white or brown

¼ cup hemp oil

5 cups water

Juice of 2 limes, about 4 tablespoons

1 ½ teaspoons fresh rosemary

¾ teaspoon chipotle

SOUP TOPPINGS

1 cup baby spinach

1 cup broccoli florets, broken into tiny pieces

½ cup cherry tomatoes, halved

¼ cup hemp nuts

Blend avocados, miso, oil, water, lime juice, rosemary, and chipotle until smooth.

To serve, place spinach leaves in bottom of four soup bowls. Pour soup base into bowls. Top each with remaining soup toppings. Serve immediately.

Toppings will keep for two days, and soup base will keep one day in the fridge when stored separately.

HOME-STYLE MINESTRONE SOUP

MAKES 4 SERVINGS

SOUP BASE

1 cup sun-dried tomatoes
2 cups water
3 stalks celery, roughly chopped
2 cloves garlic
¼ to ½ teaspoon cayenne
1 teaspoon sea salt
3 cups tomato, diced

SOUP TOPPINGS

1 zucchini, chopped
⅓ cup basil leaves, chopped
¼ cup oregano leaves
¼ cup extra virgin olive oil
Pinch ground black pepper

Soak sun-dried tomatoes for 10 minutes in 2 cups of water, or until they soften.

Blend 2 cups of soak water from the sun-dried tomatoes with the celery, garlic, cayenne, and sea salt until smooth.

Add fresh tomatoes and soaked sun-dried tomatoes to the blender. Blend on low, making sure to leave a chunky texture, like that of a chunky marinara. This isn't supposed to be a smooth soup base.

To serve, place zucchini and herbs into four soup bowls. Pour soup into each bowl. Top with a swirl of olive oil and black pepper.

Soup base with toppings will keep for one day in the fridge.

savory sauces and dips

THESE RECIPES ALL make a great addition to other dishes. Use them as a sauce, dip, or even a dressing. Or serve alongside fresh cut veggies for your party snack platter.

SUN-DRIED TOMATO MARINARA

MAKES 4 SERVINGS

This marinara is the best-tasting marinara ever. The type of tomatoes you use will determine the final flavor of this wonderful sauce. I love heirloom tomatoes—they're full of flavor. This marinara may look like it's got a lot of ingredients, but each one adds extra dimensionality. It's totally worth any extra work, I promise.

> **2 cups tomatoes, chopped**
> **1 clove garlic**
> **1/2 cup fresh basil leaves, loosely packed**
> **1/4 cup extra virgin olive oil**
> **Juice of 1/2 lemon or lime, about 1 tablespoon**
> **1 teaspoon pitted dates**
> **1 teaspoon oregano, fresh or dried**
> **1/2 teaspoon rosemary, fresh or dried**
> **1 teaspoon sea salt**
> **3 tablespoons sun-dried tomatoes**

Blend fresh tomatoes, garlic, basil, olive oil, lemon juice, dates, oregano, rosemary, and salt until smooth. Add the sun-dried tomatoes and blend until mixed well. The sun-dried tomatoes will absorb excess moisture and make your marinara thicker.

Will keep for two days in the fridge.

GARLIC CASHEW AÏOLI

MAKES 4 SERVINGS

Juice of 1 lemon, about 2 tablespoons
2 cups cashews
3 stalks celery, coarsely chopped
⅛ yellow onion, about 2 tablespoons
2 tablespoons thyme leaves
2 cloves garlic
½ cup water, as needed

Blend lemon juice, cashews, celery, onion, thyme, and garlic until smooth and creamy, adding water only as needed.

Will keep for three days in the fridge.

MISO GRAVY

MAKES 4 SERVINGS

¼ cup miso
1 tablespoon apple cider vinegar
1 clove garlic
½ orange, peeled and seeded
⅓ cup extra virgin olive oil
2 tablespoons pitted dates

Blend miso, vinegar, garlic, orange, oil, and dates until smooth.

Will keep for four days in the fridge.

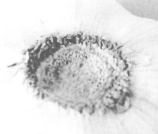

KREAMY ALMOND YOGURT

MAKES 4 SERVINGS

1 cup almonds
1 cup water, as needed
Juice of ½ lemon, about 1 tablespoon

Blend almonds and lemon juice on high to mix well in blender. Gradually add only as much water as needed to create a yogurt consistency.

To serve, use immediately or ferment.

OPTIONAL: To ferment, pour yogurt into a glass bowl or jar and cover with hemp or cheesecloth to allow the transfer of air. Set your jar in a warm place and allow it to heat up to about 90° to 100° F. You can test the temperature by sticking your finger in. It should be slightly warm to the touch. Let it sit for about 8 to 10 hours, then taste for tartness. You may need to leave it a couple more hours and taste again; repeat until it begins to taste tart.

You can also take the easy way like I do by adding 1/2 teaspoon of probiotic powder into the blender with the yogurt. The heat from the blending helps the probiotic turn the kream into instant yogurt.

Make your own flavored yogurts by adding a little lemon juice, vanilla, and your favorite fruit or fruit syrup before serving.

Will keep for three to four days in the fridge, and will continue to get more and more tart over time. You can use a couple tablespoons of overly tart yogurt in your next batch to help start the fermentation process.

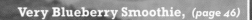
Very Blueberry Smoothie, *(page 46)*

Cherry Malt Smoothie
(page 51)

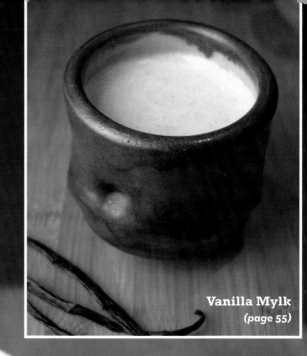

Vanilla Mylk
(page 55)

Chocolate Mylk
(page 56)

Goji Berry Sunshine Cereal
(page 67)

Fruit Parfait
(page 75)

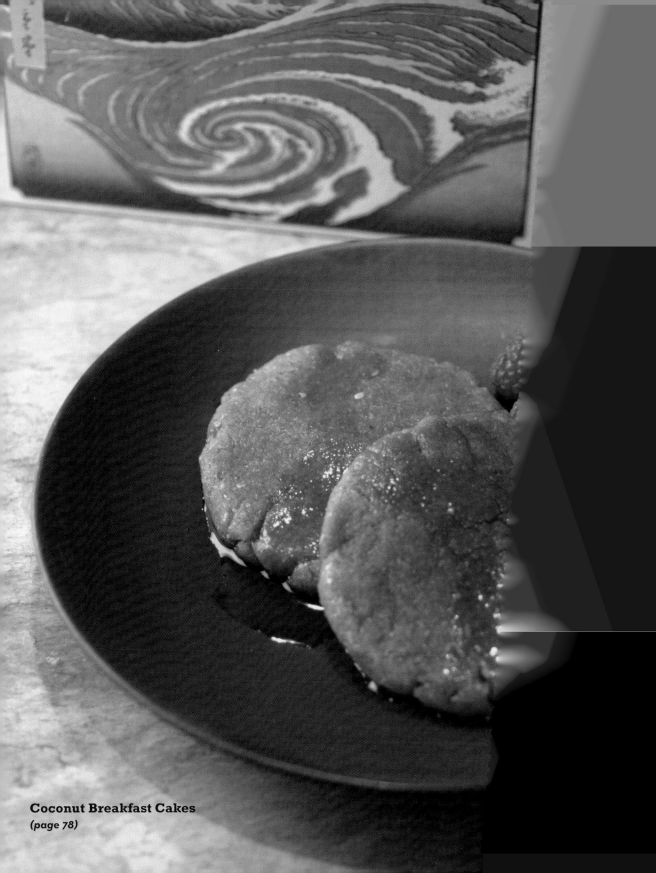

Coconut Breakfast Cakes
(page 78)

Spanish Scramble
(page 82)

Confetti Salad in Orange-Cucumber Dressing
(page 95)

Sweet Corn Chowder
(page 122)

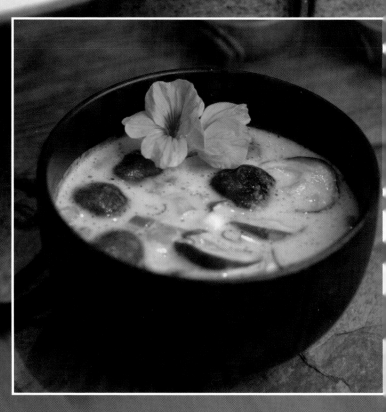

**Japanese
Miso-Shiitake Soup**
(page 118)

Walnut Cranberry Squash "Rice"

(page 140)

**Sun Burgers on Black Sesame
Sunflower Bread with
Sun-Dried Tomato Catsup**

(page 194)

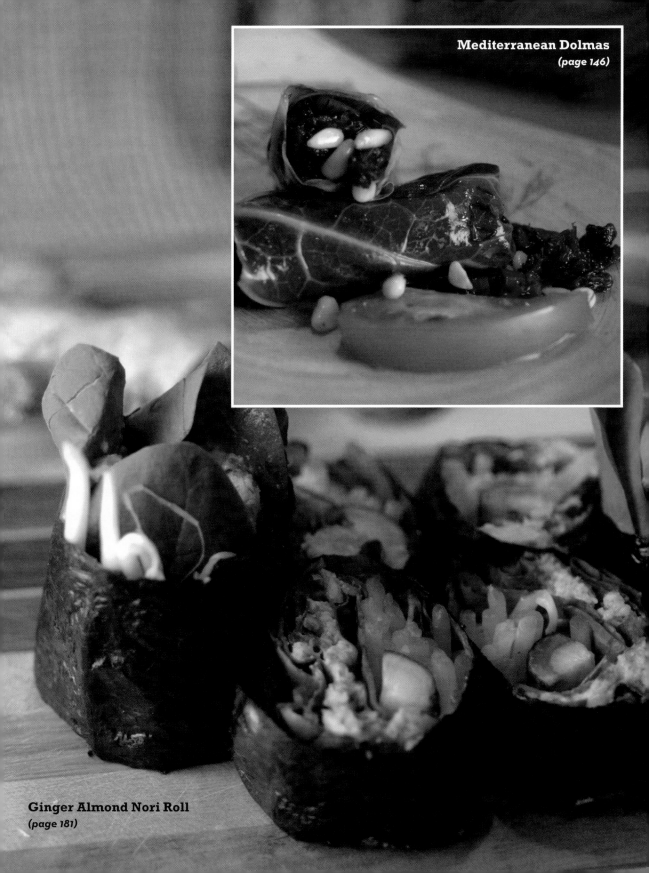

Mediterranean Dolmas
(page 146)

Ginger Almond Nori Roll
(page 181)

Stuffed Anaheim Chilies
with Mole Sauce
(page 192)

**Marinated Portabello Steak & Brazil -Broccoli Mash
with Mushroom Gravy**

(page 196)

Coco Kream Pie with Carob Fudge on Brownie Crust

(page 217)

Fresh Mango Cobbler
(page 215)

Coconut Snow Cake
(page 220)

TZATZIKI—CUCUMBERS IN YOGURT

MAKES 4 SERVINGS

1 cucumber, peeled, diced
1 teaspoon sea salt
1 cup Kreamy Almond Yogurt (page 128)
1 garlic clove, minced
¼ cup dill, chopped

Place cucumber in a strainer and set over a bowl. Toss with ½ teaspoon sea salt. Let excess water drain off for a few minutes.

Place drained cucumbers in a bowl. Add yogurt, garlic, ½ teaspoon salt, and dill. Mix well.

Will keep for one day in the fridge.

SUN-DRIED TOMATO CATSUP

MAKES 4 SERVINGS

1 tomato, diced, about 1 ½ cups
3 tablespoons pitted dates
¼ cup extra virgin olive oil
1 teaspoon sea salt
1 tablespoon apple cider vinegar
½ cup sun-dried tomatoes

Blend fresh tomato, dates, oil, salt, and vinegar until smooth. Add sun-dried tomatoes last, and blend until catsup is thick and well mixed.

Will keep for four days in the fridge.

HOT MUSTARD SAUCE

MAKES 4 SERVINGS

1 tablespoon pitted dates, or 1 tablespoon agave, maple syrup, or honey
4 tablespoons dry mustard
2 tablespoons filtered water
2 tablespoons apple cider vinegar
Juice of 1 lemon, about 2 tablespoons
Pinch turmeric
1 cup extra virgin olive oil

If using dates, begin by soaking dates in 2 tablespoons of water. Use a fork to puree into a thick syrup.

In a mixing bowl, add date syrup, mustard, water, vinegar, lemon juice, and turmeric. Stir until well blended. Slowly whisk in the olive oil until emulsified. Refrigerate, covered, until needed.

Will keep for four days in the fridge.

FERMENTED FOODS

Raw fermented foods increase healthy flora in the intestinal tract by creating the right type of environment for them to flourish. Fermented foods help break down and assimilate proteins and have a soothing effect on the nervous system. They increase our overall nutrition and support our immune function by increasing B vitamins (even vitamin B_{12}), omega 3 fatty acids, digestive enzymes, lactase and lactic acid, and other immune chemicals that fight off harmful bacteria and even cancer cells.

Fermented foods include yogurt, kombucha tea, sauerkraut, miso, olives, and pickles. Fermented Kreamy Almond Yogurt (page 128) is full of vitamin B_{12} and acidophilus, which is great for digestion.

Enjoying my favorite kombucha tea in ginger flavor from High Country. An acquired taste, this brand is potent and shifts my body's pH to be more alkaline. Besides helping me digest, it gives me energy and helps me feel good.

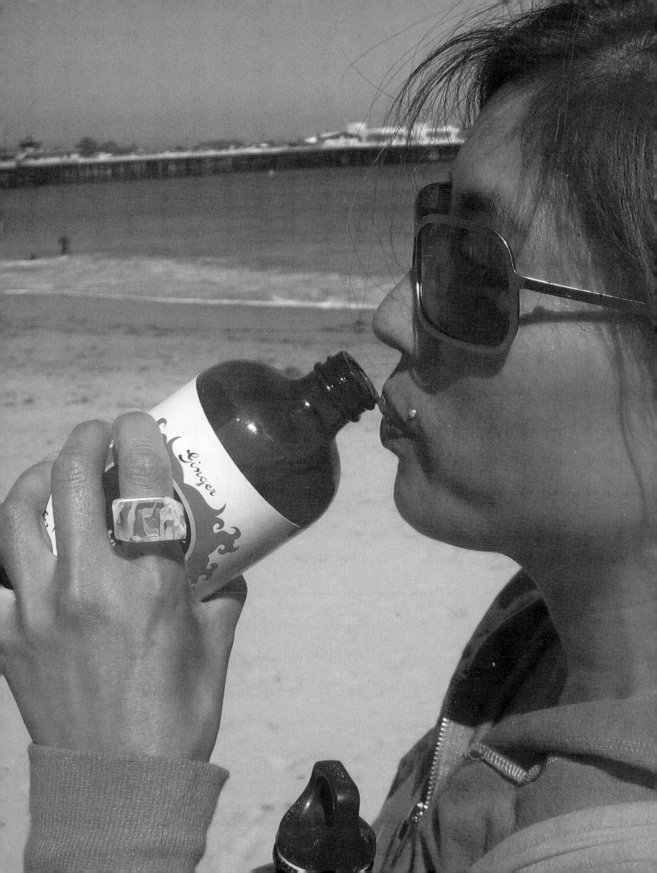

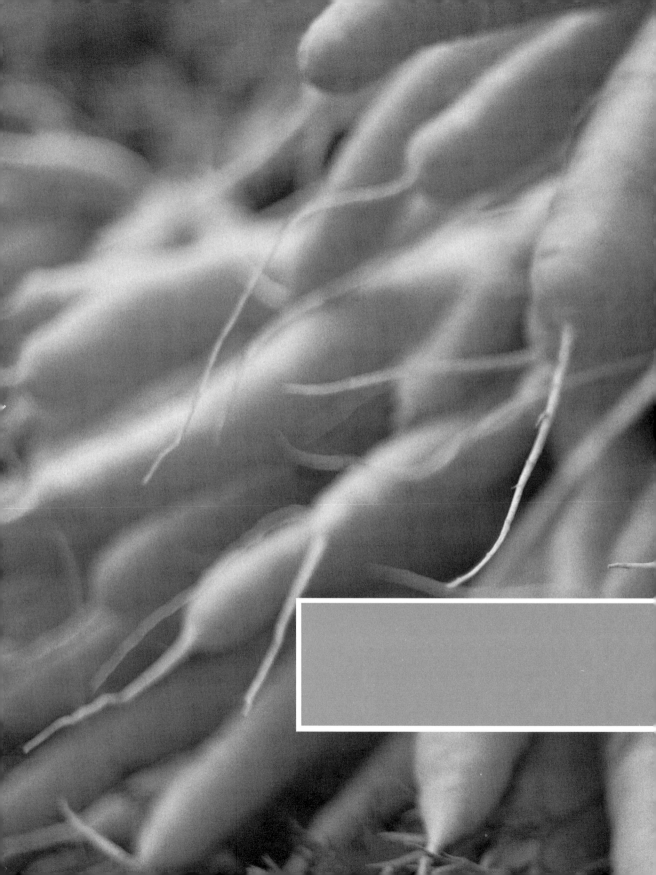

5

accompaniments and **sides**

water is life

OUR PLANET IS 70 to 80 percent water. Even our bodies are made up of 70 to 80 percent water. So it makes sense we should consume the highest quality water available. Just like us, produce is also made up of 70 to 80 percent water, and its water's been naturally distilled and filtered by the plant. It's *living* water, and it's easy for our body to absorb and use.

Think about this. In nature, water never stands still, unlike the water on our grocery shelves that sits static in plastic bottles. The rivers and ponds are alive and dynamic. When eating cooked or dehydrated foods, it's really important to hydrate our bodies as much as possible. The best way to hydrate is always through a diet high in fresh water-rich produce, where living water comes directly from the leaves and fruits of plants. These plants naturally distill mineral-rich water from deep in our earth. This living water is very different from water that comes in a plastic bottle. Beware . . . chemicals are known to leach out of the plastic bottle into the water it holds. Plus, those water bottles fill up our landfills like crazy, and take forever to break down.

ARE YOU HYDRATED?

It's a good rule of thumb to drink eight glasses of water a day to keep healthy. Water helps transport nutrients, regulates our body's temperature, aids digestion, keeps our joints supple, cleans out our body, and keeps our skin healthy and young. Water helps us maximize fat metabolism by helping our liver metabolize fat. Water is the most important nutrient for anyone who exercises; it's important to drink water before, during, and after workouts.

A way to tell if you're taking in enough water is by checking the color of your urine. It should be a pale yellow or have almost no color when you're hydrated enough.

Since water is the basis of all things living, I choose to consume fresh whole foods and living water. It's important to drink a lot of water when eating dehydrated and cooked foods, to replace the water that's missing.

HYDRATION TIPS

Everyone needs eight to ten cups of water a day, and at least ten to twelve if you're more active.

- Don't hydrate with caffeinated drinks or alcohol; they're both diuretics and dehydrating.

- Drink water throughout the day and before you get thirsty.

- Carry water bottles with you to work, on errands, and when working out.

- Notice signs of dehydration such as fatigue, headache, loss of appetite, heat intolerance, light-headedness, dry cough, dark urine, and even muscle cramps.

- When exercising, drink at least:
  two cups before working out
  one cup every twenty minutes while working out
  At least two cups of water for each pound lost after exercising

- Beware of sports drinks that contain sugar and artificial colors and flavors. Opt for electrolytes from fresh Thai baby coconuts instead.

GIVE ME CLEAN WATER

Our tap water contains chlorine, fluoride, minerals, pesticides, heavy metals, and nitrates, to name a few. According to researchers around the world, chlorine in tap water results in cancer and many other diseases. A Norwegian study of 141,000 births over a three-year period found the risk of birth defects increased 14 percent in areas with chlorinated water. Scientists have already found a link between chlorine and an increased risk of bowel, kidney, and bladder cancer. A study in Ontario funded by Health Canada found that 14 to 16 percent of bladder cancers in Ontario showed a direct correlation to drinking water containing high levels of chlorine.

One way to ensure you're drinking clean water is to look for the purest spring water sources in your region. Another is to place filters on your tap and on icemakers.

Two filtration systems to consider are reverse osmosis or solid block carbon. Both remove chlorine. Reverse osmosis removes fluoride along with many minerals good for our bones, teeth, and heart. But it wastes four to nine gallons to get one gallon of pure water. Solid block carbon filters get rid of pretty much everything but fluoride and minerals, and are so dense they don't allow the growth of bacteria within the filter.

Also think about adding a shower filter to your shower head. The American Chemical Society estimates "we could receive from 6 to 100 times more chlorine by breathing the air around showers and baths than we could by drinking water." So not only is chlorine absorbed through our skin while showering, but it also vaporizes and is inhaled into our lungs and transferred directly into our blood system.

You'll notice the more fresh produce you enjoy, the more hydrated you'll feel. When I'm thirsty, along with drinking water, I'll bite into a juicy melon or orange to hydrate myself.

COCONUTS ARE LIVING WATER

Coconut water is living water. Mineralized water from deep within the earth is sucked up by the roots of the palm tree, filtered up its trunk, and perfectly sealed inside a coconut. It takes the palm tree nine months to filter one liter of water up its trunk.

Coconuts are a great source of electrolytes. So they're a good thing to drink after a workout. I'll reach for a nutritious coconut thirst quencher over an artificially colored neon plastic bottle of sports drink any day.

The Food and Agricultural Organization of the United Nations' Chief of Agricultural Industries and Post Harvest Management Service says, "Coconut water is a natural isotonic beverage with the same level of electrolytic balance as we have in our blood. It's the fluid of life, so to speak." With the help of an Italian food technologist, they developed a cold sterilization processing method to bottle coconut water without losing the flavor and nutritional characteristic. However, I still opt for the fresh source from the whole coconut.

Plus, coconuts are the perfect glass; its water can be enjoyed directly from the husk with a straw. Dry your husks in the sun for several days. Once they're dry, they make great firewood!

And another tidbit: during World War II, doctors discovered the water in young coconuts could be used as a substitute for blood plasma, because it's sterile, cool, easily absorbed by the body, and doesn't destroy red blood cells. Coconut water is amazing—yum!

The recipes in this section make great appetizers, sides, and accompaniments to any other recipe in this book. And as with all other recipes, these call for the freshest ingredients, full of distilled living water to help keep us hydrated and healthy. As rice is a grain, my "rice" recipes instead use processed squash for its flavor and texture. Plus, it looks just like rice pieces. You'll be surprised at how little you'll miss conventional rice.

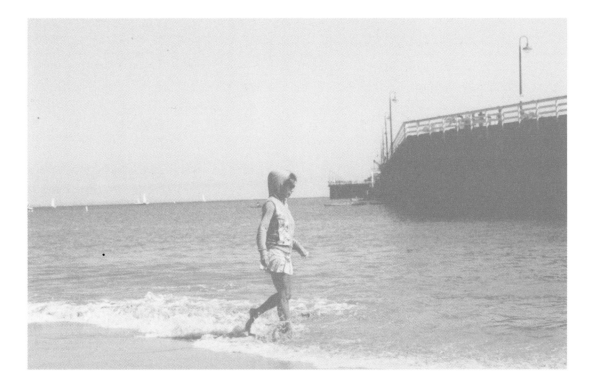

COCONUT CHUTNEY

MAKES 4 SERVINGS

Packed with electrolytes, this chutney is a great addition to any dish. Try it alongside the Walnut Cranberry Squash "Rice" (page 140) or with one of the rolls or wraps in the Moreish Mains section.

Coconut meat from 2 to 3 Thai baby coconuts, chopped, about 1 cup
Juice of 1/2 lemon, about 1 tablespoon
1 clove garlic, minced
1 small Thai red chili pepper
1/2 cup cilantro leaves, chopped
1/4 cup yellow onion, chopped
1/2 teaspoon sea salt

Blend 1/4 cup coconut meat with lemon juice.

Put coconut mixture, remaining coconut meat, garlic, chili, cilantro, onion, and salt in a bowl. Mix well.

Will keep for two days in the fridge.

Opening and Scraping a Young Thai Coconut

Please make sure never to touch or hold a coconut while cutting it. Not to scare you, but I have a friend with a scar from many stitches on her wrist. She was holding a coconut, and the knife bounced off and cut her wrist. She even drove herself to the emergency room! What a champ.

Never let children open a coconut. Be mindful and extra careful. You may want to use a cheap knife or buy a cleaver dedicated to cutting coconuts.

To open your coconut, place it sitting on a chopping board. Make three cuts in a triangle formation in the top using the heel of your knife. I like to use a cleaver on my coconuts. Empty out the water, or drink with a straw.

To cut your coconut in half, place on a chopping board. Without touching or holding the coconut, hit it hard with your cleaver through the center several times until it splits in half.

To scrape your coconut, use a large strong spoon to get under the coconut meat and to work it away from the husk.

To clean your coconut meat, run your fingers over the meat. Pick off any hard husk. Anything that's soft to the touch is okay to leave. You may want to give the meat a final rinse with water to clean it.

Will keep for two to three days in the fridge.

Optional: Try coating your coconut meat with a couple tablespoons of Nama Shoyu and olive oil, then dehydrate at 104°F for 4 to 6 hours to make a Coconut Jerky that'll keep for a week, if it doesn't all get eaten up before then!

WALNUT CRANBERRY SQUASH "RICE"

MAKES 4 SERVINGS

Cranberries are packed with antioxidants and promote a healthy heart, teeth, gums, and urinary tract. They help fight cancer and may help prevent stomach ulcers.

Use plain dried cranberries or cranberries sweetened with juice instead of sugar. If cranberries are hard to find, you can also use raisins or dates instead.

Enjoy Walnut Cranberry Squash "Rice" as a main dish with Coconut Chutney (page 138) and a soup or salad. Or try it with Save-the-Salmon Patties with Hollandaise Sauce (page 193).

1 small butternut squash, about 1 pound, peeled, seeded, and cut into 2-inch cubes
½ small yellow onion, about ½ cup, chopped
1 tablespoon cumin seeds
1 tablespoon coriander powder
½ cup cilantro leaves, chopped
1 cup dried cranberries
1 cup walnuts, crushed
2 teaspoons sea salt

Put small batches of cubed squash in a food processor and process into small pieces.

Put processed squash in a large mixing bowl. Add onion, cumin, coriander, cilantro, cranberries, walnut, and salt and mix well.

Will keep for two days in the fridge.

ANI'S KITCHEN TIP

Peeling Squash

A potato peeler works great for peeling the skin off squash. Once peeled, cut squash in half lengthwise and remove the seeds. Then cut it into smaller pieces.

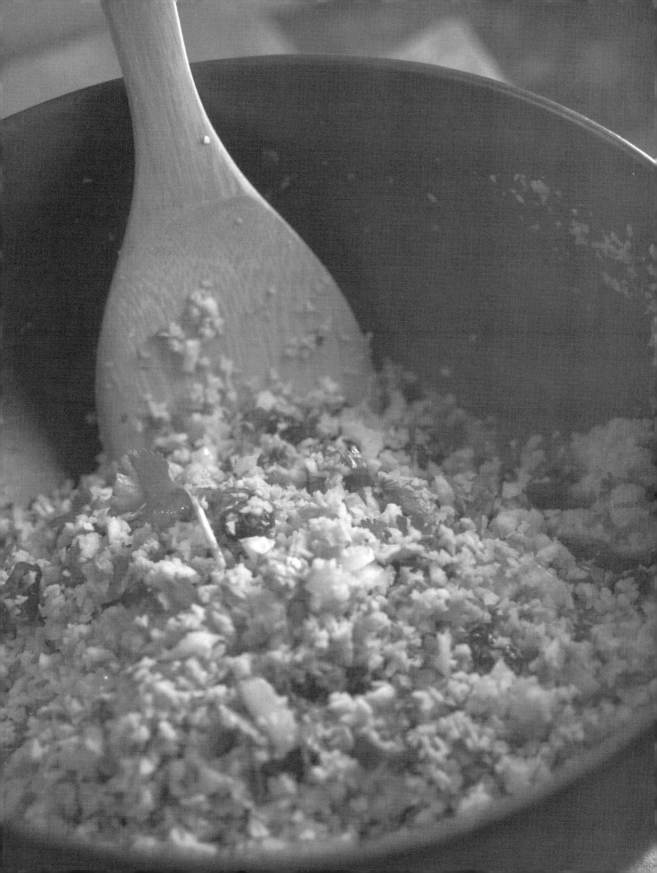

MEXICAN SQUASH "RICE"

MAKES 4 SERVINGS

Enjoy with Stuffed Anaheim Chili with Mole Sauce (page 192) or Baja Cheeze Burrito with Taco Nut Meat and Red Pepper Corn Salsa (page 189).

> **1 acorn squash, about 1 pound, peeled, seeded, and cut into 2-inch cubes**
> **1 large tomato, seeded and chopped**
> **2 tablespoons yellow onion, chopped**
> **1 clove garlic, minced**
> **¼ cup cilantro leaves, chopped**
> **1 teaspoon sea salt**

Put small batches of cubed squash in a food processor and process into small pieces.

Put processed squash in a large mixing bowl. Add tomato, onion, garlic, cilantro, and salt and mix well.

Will keep for two days in the fridge.

THAI-STYLE CUCUMBERS

MAKES 4 SERVINGS

Enjoy with Pad Thai Noodles in Almond Kaffir Sauce (page 186) or Mushroom Risotto with White Truffle–Infused Olive Oil (page 188).

> **3 cucumbers, peeled and thinly sliced**
> **1 teaspoon sea salt**
> **3 tablespoons basil chiffonade (page 120)**
> **½ tablespoon minced ginger**
> **Juice of 2 limes, about 4 tablespoons**
> **2 to 3 red chilies, seeded and finely chopped**

Toss cucumbers with salt. Let sit for about 10 minutes. Strain off excess water and toss cucumbers with basil, ginger, lime juice, and chilies. Serve immediately.

BRAZIL-BROCCOLI MASH

MAKES 4 SERVINGS

This mash is one of my favorite dishes, and really does have the mashed potato texture to it. It's really yummy. I enjoy this on its own all the time. Enjoy with Miso Gravy (page 127).

> **1 clove garlic**
> **1 pinch ground black pepper**
> **1 teaspoon sea salt**
> **1 cup Brazil nuts**
> **2 cups broccoli, chopped**

Process the garlic, pepper, and salt into tiny pieces. Add Brazil nuts and process into a powder. Empty this powder into a bowl and set aside. Next, process broccoli while slowly adding the Brazil nut powder back in.

CAULIFLOWER MISO MASH

MAKES 4 SERVINGS

This mash is thickened using psyllium powder. It has a great flavor, and it's delicious on its own too. Enjoy with Miso Gravy (page 127).

> **1 clove garlic**
> **1 head cauliflower, chopped**
> **2 tablespoons white miso**
> **1/2 cup extra virgin olive oil**
> **Juice of 1 lemon, about 2 tablespoons**
> **1 1/2 teaspoons psyllium powder**
> **1 teaspoon poultry seasoning**

Process garlic into small pieces. Add the cauliflower in small batches and process. Add remaining ingredients and process until smooth.

INDIAN-SPICED CASHEWS

MAKES 4 SERVINGS

This makes a great travel snack. It's yummy added to salads, especially those iceberg or romaine salads from restaurants when eating out.

> **1 cup cashews, soaked at least 8 hours in water, rinsed well**
> **1 tablespoon garam masala**
> **¼ teaspoon sea salt**

Put cashews still wet from soaking and rinsing in a bowl. Coat with garam marsala and sea salt.

Place coated cashews on dehydrator trays. Dehydrate at 104º F for 4 to 6 hours, or until dry.

Non-dehydrated cashews will keep three days in the fridge. Dehydrated cashews will keep for a week or more.

NO-DEHYDRATION OPTION: You can instead coat cashews in 2 tablespoons of olive oil first. Then coat with garam masala and sea salt, and serve immediately.

SWEET SPICED PECANS

MAKES 4 SERVINGS

This also makes a great travel snack. It adds extra flavor and nutrients to salads, especially those iceberg or romaine salads from restaurants when eating out.

¼ cup pitted dates, or ¼ cup agave, maple syrup, or honey
¼ teaspoon sea salt
¼ teaspoon cayenne powder
¼ teaspoon cardamom powder
Pinch of nutmeg powder
1 cup pecan halves

If using dates, soak them in ¼ cup of water for 5 to 10 minutes, or until soft. Mash dates with water until it is a thick syrup.

Put syrup, salt, cayenne, cardamom, and nutmeg in a bowl. Mix well. Add pecan halves to syrup mixture. Mix well, making sure each pecan is coated. Enjoy immediately.

OPTIONAL: Dehydrate pecans at 104º F for 4 to 6 hours, until dry.

Non-dehydrated pecans will keep two days in the fridge. Dehydrated pecans will keep for a week or more.

MEDITERRANEAN DOLMAS

MAKES 4 SERVINGS

Enjoy as a main dish with Sun-Dried Tomato Hummus (page 148), or as an appetizer before the Mushroom Risotto with White Truffle–Infused Olive Oil (page 188) or Polenta with Mushroom Ragout (page 190).

FILLING

½ cup sun-dried tomatoes, sliced
¼ cup dill, chopped
¼ cup raisins
½ cup pine nuts
2 tablespoons extra virgin olive oil
Pinch sea salt

"VINE LEAF" WRAPPER

1 collard leaf

To make filling, soak sliced sun-dried tomatoes in 1 cup of water for 10 minutes until soft. Mix dill, raisins, nuts, oil, and salt. Add softened sun-dried tomatoes and mix well.

To make "vine leaf" wrapper, cut collard leaf from stem. Cut leaf in half again so you have four pieces.

Fill each wrapper with a quarter of the filling. Fold down top and bottom edges, rotate 90 degrees and roll up.

Will keep for two days in the fridge.

PER SERVING: calories 220, protein 4g, carbohydrate 13g, fat 16g, sugar 7g
PERCENT DAILY VALUES: potassium 12%, vitamin A 4%, vitamin C 6%, calcium 2%, iron 10%, vitamin E 8%, thiamin 7%, riboflavin 5%, niacin 7%, vitamin B6 3%, folate 3%, vitamin K 28%, phosphorus 13%, magnesium 15%, zinc 8%, copper 18%, manganese 84%, dietary fiber 7%

CASHEW SOUR KREAM AND CHIVES

MAKES 4 SERVINGS

A ¼-cup dollop of Sour Kream is always a great addition on top of a soup and with Stuffed Anaheim Chilies (page 192).

1 cup cashews
Juice from 1 lemon, about 2 tablespoons
Pinch sea salt
¼ cup water, as needed
2 tablespoons chives, chopped

Blend cashews, lemon juice, salt, and just enough water to blend into a smooth kream.

Put sour kream in a bowl and stir in chopped chives.

Will keep for four days in the fridge.

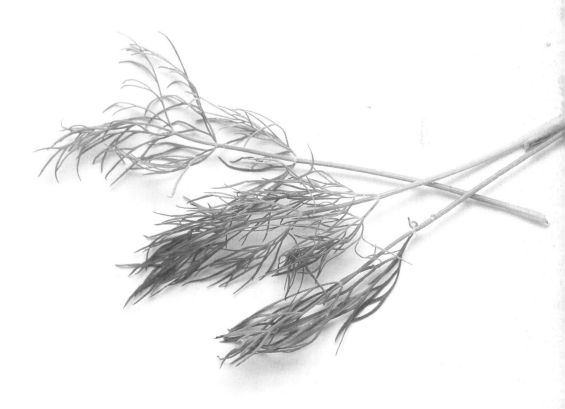

SUN-DRIED TOMATO HUMMUS (BEAN-FREE)

MAKES 4 SERVINGS

You know the old adage "beans, beans, they're good for your heart," but they give us gas. Ever wonder why? It's because our body lacks an enzyme to split their sugar, which is a disaccharide, or double sugar. Because this sugar is not fully digested, it travels through the digestive system to the bowel, ferments, and creates gas. Overcooking beans breaks the sugar bond and reduces the production of gas, but much of the nutritional value is lost.

I stay away from raw legumes in general, because I find them hard to digest. I created this alternative bean-free hummus recipe instead.

Serve with cabbage leaves cut into triangles, like chips, or with cut vegetables like broccoli, carrots, celery. Or serve with Mediterranean Dolmas (page 146) or any of the wraps or rolls in the Moreish Mains section.

2 cups zucchini, chopped
2 cloves garlic
Juice of 1 lemon, about 2 tablespoons
¼ cup plus 1 tablespoon extra virgin olive oil
½ cup tahini
1 teaspoon sea salt
2 tablespoons parsley leaves, chopped
⅓ cup sun-dried tomatoes, chopped
Pinch paprika

Process zucchini, garlic, lemon juice, ¼ cup olive oil, tahini, and salt until smooth. Pour mixture into a bowl, and stir in parsley and sun-dried tomatoes. Set aside and allow sun-dried tomatoes to soak up moisture for about 10 minutes or more. Stir well.

Sprinkle a pinch of paprika and drizzle with a tablespoon of olive oil just before serving.

Will keep for two days in the fridge.

BLACK OLIVE HUMMUS (BEAN-FREE)

MAKES 4 SERVINGS

This is another disaccharide-free hummus, which is much easier to digest and tastes amazing!

Serve with Baja Cheeze Burrito with Taco Nut Meat and Red Pepper Corn Salsa (page 189) or Black Sesame Sunflower Bread (page 153).

> **⅓ cup sunflower seeds, dried**
> **2 cups zucchini, chopped**
> **2 cloves garlic**
> **Juice of 1 lemon, about 2 tablespoons**
> **¼ cup plus 1 tablespoon extra virgin olive oil**
> **½ cup tahini**
> **¼ cup kalamata black olives, pitted and chopped**
> **Pinch paprika**

Process sunflower seeds into a powder. Set aside. Process zucchini, garlic, lemon juice, ¼ cup olive oil, and tahini until smooth. Slowly add sunflower powder back into food processor. Process until mixture reaches a smooth hummus consistency.

Pour mixture into a bowl and stir in chopped black olives. Sprinkle with paprika and drizzle with remaining olive oil.

Will keep for three days in the fridge.

PISTACHIO PESTO

MAKES 4 SERVINGS

My good friend Dawn makes some amazingly delicious pesto, and she inspired me to create this recipe.

Enjoy this pesto with Black Sesame Sunflower Bread (page 153), cut vegetables like carrots and cauliflower, or tossed with spiralized squash for Angel-Hair Squash Pasta in Pesto Sauce (page 183).

2 cloves garlic
1 teaspoon sea salt
2 cups pistachios
4 cups basil leaves, lightly packed, about 2 bunches
Juice of 3 limes, about 6 tablespoons
1/2 cup extra virgin olive oil

Process garlic, salt, and pistachios into powder. Set aside. Pulse basil with lime juice. Add pistachio meal back into processor with olive oil. Process until mixed well.

Will keep for three days in the fridge.

ROSEMARY GUACAMOLE

MAKES 4 SERVINGS

Serve with any wrap or roll from the Moreish Mains chapter. Or put a 1/4 cup scoop on top of any salad.

2 avocados, diced
2 tablespoons yellow onion, chopped
1 tablespoon fresh rosemary, chopped
Juice of 1 lemon, about 2 tablespoons
2 tablespoons extra virgin olive oil
1/2 jalapeño pepper, chopped, to taste

Put avocados, onion, rosemary, lemon juice, olive oil, and jalapeño in a bowl and mix well.

Will keep for one day in the fridge.

RED PEPPER CORN SALSA

MAKES 4 SERVINGS

Enjoy in Baja Cheeze Burrito with Taco Nut Meat and Red Pepper Corn Salsa (page 189) or scooped onto your favorite soup base.

> ½ cup red bell pepper, chopped
> 1 cup corn kernels, cut from the cob
> ½ cup tomatoes, diced
> ½ cup cilantro leaves, chopped
> ¼ cup scallions, chopped
> 1 clove garlic, minced
> ½ jalapeño pepper, chopped
> 1 teaspoon sea salt

Mix bell pepper, corn, tomatoes, cilantro, scallions, garlic, jalapeño, and salt in a bowl.

Will keep for one day in the fridge.

CASHEW GARLIC PARMESAN SPRINKLE

MAKES 4 SERVINGS

Use this sprinkle to top salads, pastas, and soups. It really reminds me of dairy parmesan cheese.

> 1 clove garlic
> ½ teaspoon sea salt
> 1 cup cashews

Process garlic and salt. Add cashews and process into a powder.

Will keep for four days in the fridge.

ASPARAGUS WITH CHEEZY SAUCE

MAKES 4 SERVINGS

ASPARAGUS
- 1 bunch asparagus
- ½ teaspoon sea salt
- 2 tablespoons extra virgin olive oil

CHEEZY SAUCE
- 2 cloves garlic
- 1 teaspoon sea salt
- 1 cup sunflower seeds
- Juice of 1 lemon, about 2 tablespoons
- 1 teaspoon turmeric
- ¼ cup water, as needed

To prepare asparagus, trim off the bottom inch of each stalk. Cut the thicker stalks in half. Toss in sea salt and olive oil, and set aside.

To make sauce, process garlic and salt until smooth. Add sunflower seeds and process into a powder. Add lemon juice and turmeric and mix well. Gradually add just enough water for a creamy cheesy sauce texture.

To serve, place asparagus on four plates. Drizzle Cheezy Sauce over each.

OPTIONAL: You can dehydrate asparagus at 104° F for 1 hour. Don't over-dehydrate; you just want to help the asparagus wilt and soften a bit. Serve warm with Cheezy Sauce drizzled on top.

Will keep for two days in the fridge.

BLACK SESAME SUNFLOWER BREAD

MAKES 4 TO 5 SERVINGS

This is a great "bread" to use as morning toast, as a base for pizzas, and as a "bun" for sun burgers. The recipe calls for black sesame seeds, but tan seeds will work fine, too.

I under-dehydrate bread for immediate use, so some of the water still remains. The bread is more pliable that way. It'll keep in your fridge for several days, but you'll want to fully dehydrate the bread before storing it away for longer periods of time.

This recipe will fill one Excalibur dehydrator tray, and yields nine slices of bread. I recommend tripling or quadrupling your batch. It'll keep for at least a month or two when fully dried. Keep refrigerated.

This bread travels really well. I like to take it on trips with me, and just buy an avocado and make sandwiches on the road. Or serve immediately and warm with butter or a burger.

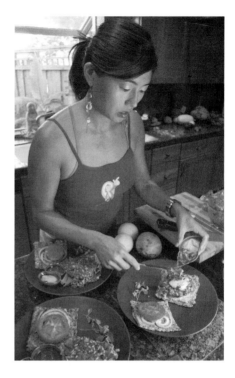

1 cup ground flax seeds

1/3 cup whole flax seeds

1/2 teaspoon sea salt

1 clove garlic, minced

2 tablespoons yellow onion, chopped

1 1/3 cups water

2/3 cup sunflower seeds

1/4 cup black sesame seeds

Mix ground and whole flax seeds, salt, garlic, onion, and water. Add sunflower and sesame seeds and and mix well.

Use the back of a spoon to spread batter evenly on one dehydrator tray. Dry at 104° F for 4 hours. Flip and score bread into nine slices to make it easy to break in straight lines. Dehydrate another hour before serving. Serve warm.

BLACK SESAME SUNFLOWER CROUTONS

MAKES ABOUT 10 SERVINGS

Follow the recipe for Black Sesame Sunflower Bread (page 153). When flipping bread in dehydrator, score into 1-inch squares. Dehydrate another hour and serve warm. Enjoy as you would toasted croutons on salads and in soups. Great in wraps, too!

Make extra to keep on hand. Dehydrate fully before storing. Will keep for at least a month or two.

TACO NUT MEAT

MAKES 4 SERVINGS

Use this taco nut meat like you would regular non-vegan taco meat. Top salads, make a wrap, or add it in a burrito. It adds a kick of instantly rich flavor.

> **½ cup almonds, dry**
> **½ cup walnuts, dry**
> **1 tablespoon ground cumin**
> **1 tablespoon ground coriander**
> **⅓ cup extra virgin olive oil**
> **⅔ teaspoon sea salt**
> **1 teaspoon Nama Shoyu or Bragg Liquid Aminos**

Process almonds and walnuts into a powder.

Place nut meal into a mixing bowl. Add cumin, coriander, olive oil, salt, and Nama Shoyu and mix well.

Will keep for four days in the fridge.

BLACK OLIVE TAPENADE

MAKES 4 SERVINGS

Tapenade is a rich olive spread popular in the Mediterranean. It's quite easy to make at home.

Measure out 1 cup of olives first. Then pit them. Olives are easy to pit if you just push down onto a cutting board from above with your fingers around the pit. Rub the oil from the olives into your skin as a natural hand moisture treatment.

Serve with Black Sesame Sunflower Bread (page 153) and with any pasta recipe from the Moreish Mains chapter.

> 1 clove garlic
> 1 cup black olives, pitted
> Juice of ½ lemon, about 1 tablespoon
> 2 tablespoons extra virgin olive oil
> 1 tablespoon thyme, fresh or dried
> 2 teaspoons rosemary, fresh or dried

Process garlic into small pieces. Put lemon juice, olive oil, thyme, and rosemary in processor and pulse to combine well. Allow to process until mix is coarsely pureed.

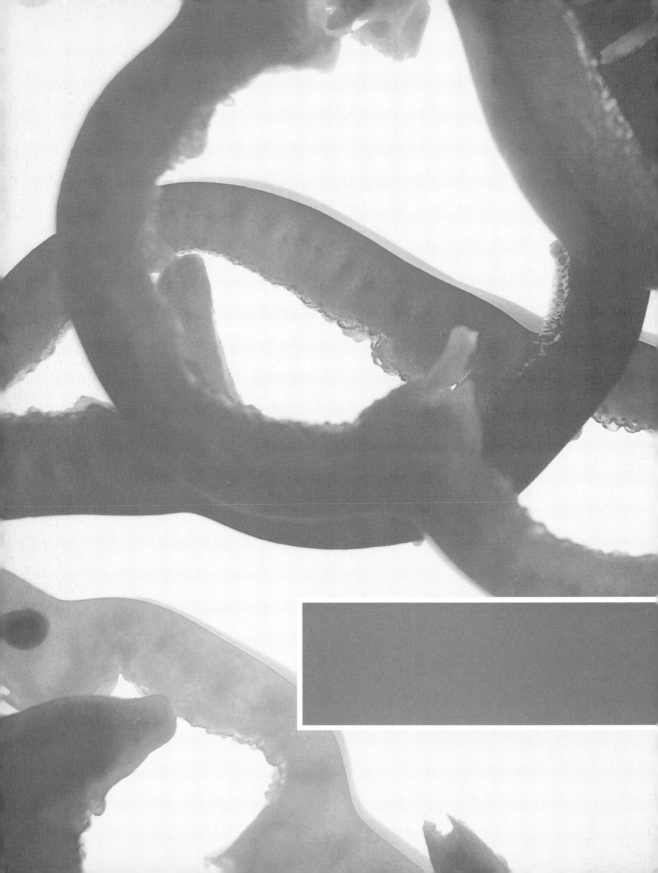

6

scrumptious **cheezes**
and **pâtés**

live toxic-free

TOXIC-FREE LIVING involves much more than just eating organic food. The most poisonous place in many homes is under the kitchen sink—where most people store their chemical cleansers. Chemicals in household cleansers can be toxic—in fact, according to the EPA, some of the most common ones are three times more likely to cause cancer than outdoor air pollution!

Have you noticed as you walk through the grocery store you can often smell the cleaning aisle before you even get there? This is because chemicals outgas through their plastic containers, meaning the toxic vapors pass through the plastic containers and into the air. If you can smell it, it's in the air, in your environment, and in your lungs. Whether chemicals are used to clean in your environment or just sit under your bathroom or kitchen sink, the vapors are still getting into your environment and into your lungs. And once you use these chemicals, they wash down our sinks and into our water supply.

Other things emit toxic chemicals, too. Toxic chemicals used when making carpets, for example, are brought into our homes and continue to emit formaldehyde (H_2CO) gas. And most of the paints used on walls are toxic, giving off volatile organic compounds (VOCs). Try to use only natural cleansers, which are safest for your health and won't damage our environment.

LEMON RINDS ARE GREAT FOR CLEANING AND DEGREASING

You'll notice after you make many of the recipes in this section, you're left with lemon rinds. Many commercial cleansers add lemon to help cut grease. Go directly to the organic source: leftover citrus rinds make great cleansers. Just use the rind instead of a sponge on hard-to-clean areas.

I gather rinds from a dozen lemons, put them in my bathtub, fill it with cold water overnight, then drain and wipe clean with a sponge the next morning. My bath is left sparkling clean with very little elbow grease.

Baking soda and vinegar are great cleansers, too. Just dissolve 4 tablespoons of baking soda in 1 quart of warm water and use as a general cleanser, or use on a damp sponge to clean and deodorize all kitchen and bathroom surfaces. Use undiluted vinegar to remove stubborn hard water spots and streaks on glass.

BATHING

Try using organic natural soaps, shampoos, conditioners, and toothpaste. They don't contain toxic chemicals that eventually wash down our drain and into our water supply. So it's important they're not harmful for us.

NATURAL FIBERS

Synthetic and nonorganic fibers go through chemical processing. As a result, those chemicals stay in the fabric. When you have it against your skin, you're absorbing the chemicals into your body. And when it's in your environment, it emits those toxins into the air. Look for organic fabrics, such as cotton and hemp, especially for clothes, bedding, and other household items.

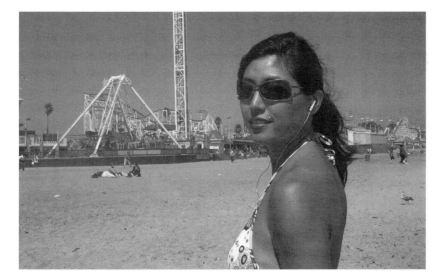

It's hard to escape air pollution. But the following things can help lower the effects: limit time spent near auto and industrial emissions, buy an air purifier, add living green plants to your home, eat antioxidant-rich foods like kale, berries, apples, and cherries.

cheezes

I USED TO love cheese, but dairy products weren't good for me or my cholesterol levels. I developed these raw cheezes to be used in the same way dairy cheeses are. They're great tasting and high in protein. My cheezes have the texture of a whipped cheese, hummus spread, or fondue dip.

Enjoy any of these cheezes in wraps, rolls, on salads, as a dip for vegetables, and on Black Sesame Sunflower Bread (page 153). Use them to stuff tomatoes and peppers and between layers of sliced squash and Sun-Dried Tomato Marinara (page 126) to make a delicious Italian Rawzania (page 185). Use them as you would any spread or hummus.

Feel free to try my cheezes in your cooked bread sandwiches as a dairy cheese substitute, too.

I always keep a batch of cheeze around. It's a great basic ingredient for fast treats. Wrap some up in a kale or cabbage leaf or in a sheet of nori, or scoop some on top of a green salad instead of using dressing. Cheezes are made with nuts, seeds, herbs, and spices.

All cheezes and spreads will last about four to five days in the fridge.

ITALIAN PIZZA CHEEZE

MAKES 4 SERVINGS

Serve with Pizza with Sun-Dried Tomatoes, Black Olives, and Fresh Italian Herbs (page 197).

>**2 cups macadamia nuts**
>**Juice of 1 lemon, about 2 tablespoons**
>**3 cloves garlic**
>**1/2 cup basil leaves**
>**1 teaspoon sea salt**
>**2/3 cup water, as needed**

Blend nuts, lemon juice, garlic, basil, and salt until smooth, adding only enough water as needed to make a smooth, creamy texture.

Will keep for four days in the fridge.

BLACK PEPPER CHEEZE

MAKES 4 SERVINGS

Enjoy with Stuffed Anaheim Chili with Mole Sauce (page 192).

>**2 cups cashews**
>**Juice of 2 lemons, about 4 tablespoons**
>**3 cloves garlic**
>**1/2 teaspoon ground black pepper**
>**1 teaspoon sea salt**
>**1/4 cup water**

Process cashews, lemon juice, garlic, pepper, and salt until smooth, adding only enough water as needed to make a smooth, creamy texture.

Will keep for four days in the fridge.

PER SERVING: calories 301, protein 10g, carbohydrate 16g, fat 24g, sugar 3g
PERCENT DAILY VALUES: potassium 12%, vitamin C 13%, calcium 4%, iron 24%, vitamin E 2%, thiamin 10%, riboflavin 8%, niacin 5%, vitamin B6 11%, folate 12%, pantothenic acid 9%, vitamin K 30%, phosphorus 34%, magnesium 45%, zinc 26%, copper 77%, manganese 31%, selenium 12%, dietary fiber 9%

CRUSHED RED PEPPER–CRUSTED CHEEZE PATTY

MAKES 4 SERVINGS

Enjoy on top of any salad and with Black Sesame Sunflower Bread (page 153).

> **1 batch of Black-Pepper Cheeze (page 161)**
> **1/2 cup crushed, dried hot red pepper flakes**

Use your hands to shape 1/2 -cup patties.

To serve, place crushed red pepper in a bowl. Roll each patty in pepper and coat all surfaces.

Will keep for four days in the fridge.

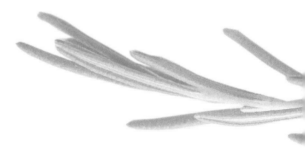

SUN-DRIED TOMATO CHEEZE

MAKES 4 SERVINGS

Enjoy as a sandwich with Black Sesame Sunflower Bread (page 153) and fresh slices of tomato and avocado.

> **2 cloves garlic**
> **1 teaspoon sea salt**
> **2 cups Brazil nuts**
> **Juice of 2 lemons, about 4 tablespoons**
> **1/2 cup water, as needed**
> **1 cup sun-dried tomatoes, chopped**

Process garlic and salt into small pieces. Add Brazil nuts and process into a powder. Add lemon juice and mix well. Gradually add only enough water as needed to make a heavy kream. Scoop kream into a bowl and mix in sun-dried tomatoes.

Will keep for four days in the fridge.

HERB-CRUSTED CHEEZE PATTY

MAKES 4 SERVINGS

Enjoy on top of any salad and with Black Sesame Sunflower Bread (page 153).

> **1 batch Sun-Dried Tomato Cheeze (page 162)**
> **1 cup fresh parsley, chopped**
> **2 tablespoons fresh rosemary, chopped**

Use your hands to shape ½ -cup patties using a very dry batch of Sun-Dried Tomato Cheeze.

Place parsley and rosemary in a bowl. Roll each patty in herbs and coat all surfaces. Serve immediately.

RICOTTA CHEEZE

MAKES 4 SERVINGS

Enjoy as a substitute for Italian Pizza Cheeze in your Italian Rawzania (page 185). Or simply serve 2 to 3 tablespoons between slices of heirloom tomatoes, and drizzle with olive oil before serving.

> **2 cloves garlic**
> **1 cup pine nuts**
> **1 cup walnuts**
> **½ cup fresh parsley**
> **⅓ cup miso**
> **Juice of 1 lemon, about 2 tablespoons**
> **1 cup water, as needed**

Process garlic into small pieces. Add pine nuts and walnuts and process into powder. Then add miso and lemon juice. Process, adding just enough water to make a chunky Ricotta Cheeze. Lastly, lightly process in fresh parsley to mix.

Will keep for four days in the fridge.

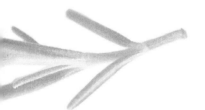

SUNNY DILL CHEEZE

MAKES 4 SERVINGS

Enjoy as the base to your Save-the-Salmon Patties with Hollandaise Sauce (page 193), or scooped onto your favorite salad.

2 cups sunflower seeds
Juice of 1 lemon, about 2 tablespoons
3 cloves garlic
1 bunch dill
1/2 cup water, as needed

Blend sunflower seeds, lemon juice, garlic, and dill until smooth, adding water as needed to make a creamy texture.

Will keep for four days in the fridge.

BAJA CHEEZE

MAKES 4 SERVINGS

Enjoy with Baja Cheeze Burrito with Taco Nut Meat and Red Pepper Corn Salsa (page 189).

2 cups Brazil nuts
Juice of 2 lemons, about 4 tablespoons
3 cloves garlic
1/2 habanero or jalapeño pepper
1 bunch cilantro leaves
1/2 cup water, as needed

Blend nuts, lemon juice, garlic, habanero, and cilantro until smooth, adding only as much water as needed to create a smooth cheeze.

Will keep for four days in the fridge.

OREGANO RICOTTA

MAKES 4 SERVINGS

Enjoy as a substitute for Italian Pizza Cheeze in your Italian Rawzania (page 185). Or simply serve 2 to 3 tablespoons between slices of heirloom tomatoes.

> **2 medium garlic cloves**
> **1 teaspoon sea salt**
> **2 cups cashews**
> **Juice of 2 lemons, about 4 tablespoons**
> **1 tablespoon extra virgin olive oil**
> **3 tablespoons oregano**
> **½ cup water, as needed**

Process garlic and salt into small pieces. Add cashews and process into a powder. Add lemon juice, olive oil, and oregano and process. Add only enough water to make a chunky Ricotta Cheeze texture.

Will keep for three days in the fridge.

NACHO CHEEZE

MAKES 4 SERVINGS

Enjoy with Black Sesame Sunflower Bread (page 153), or drizzled over cut vegetables like asparagus or broccoli.

> **2 cups macadamia nuts**
> **Juice of 2 lemons, about 4 tablespoons**
> **1 tablespoon Nama Shoyu or Bragg Liquid Aminos**
> **1 tablespoon turmeric**
> **1 to 2 teaspoons cayenne pepper**
> **1 cup water, as needed**

Process nuts, lemon juice, Nama Shoyu, turmeric, and cayenne and slowly add just enough water for desired consistency.

Will keep for three days in the fridge.

pâtés

Like cheezes, pâtés are great to keep on hand. They make a scrumptious addition to salads and can be wrapped up in nori or lettuce in a snap to feed your hunger. Pâtés are made mostly with nuts, seeds, and vegetables.

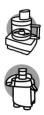

SAVE-THE-TUNA PÂTÉ

MAKES 4 SERVINGS

This is a two-part recipe. Begin with the pâté base, then stir in the "salad" bits . . . and voila! A delicious mock tuna salad, without the mercury.

Enjoy with Save-the-Tuna Wrap (page 179).

If you don't have a veggie juicer, substitute with 2 grated carrots instead.

PÂTÉ BASE

2 cloves garlic
1 tablespoon dulse flakes
2 cups sunflower seeds
Juice of 2 lemons, about 4 tablespoons
1/2 cup water, as needed

TUNA SALAD

Pulp from 1 pound washed, peeled, and juiced carrots
1/2 bunch fresh parsley leaves, chopped
1/4 cup yellow onion, chopped
1/8 teaspoon ground black pepper
2 stalks celery, chopped

To make pâté base, process garlic and dulse in food processor to chop up garlic. Then add sunflower seeds and process into a powder. Add lemon juice and just as much water as needed to make a thick kream.

Scoop the pâté base into a large bowl. Add the carrot pulp, parsley, onion, pepper, and celery and mix well.

Will keep for two days in the fridge.

GINGER ALMOND PÂTÉ

MAKES 4 SERVINGS

Enjoy with Ginger Almond Nori Roll (page 181).

> **2 tablespoons grated ginger**
> **2 cloves garlic**
> **1 teaspoon sea salt**
> **2 cups almonds**
> **Juice of 2 lemons, about 4 tablespoons**
> **½ cup water, as needed**

Process ginger, garlic, and salt until mixed well. Add almonds and process while adding lemon juice. Add water only as needed for a hummus-like texture.

Will keep for three days in the fridge.

GARDEN PÂTÉ

MAKES 4 SERVINGS

> **1 cup almonds, dry**
> **1 tablespoon grated ginger**
> **2 cloves garlic**
> **1 teaspoon sea salt**
> **3 carrots, chopped**
> **2 stalks celery, chopped**
> **¼ cup yellow onion, chopped**
> **2 tablespoons extra virgin olive oil**
> **Juice of ½ lemon, about 1 tablespoon**
> **½ cup raisins**

Process almonds into a powder. Empty into large bowl and set aside.

Next, process ginger, garlic, and sea salt to chop up the ginger and garlic. Add carrots, celery, and onion and pulse into small pieces. Add olive oil, lemon juice, raisins, and almond powder. Mix well.

Scoop ½ cup on a bed of greens, or place into a lettuce leaf to make a wrap. Or enjoy between slices of Black Sesame Sunflower Bread. (page 153).

OPTIONAL: Form ½ -cup patties and dehydrate 3 to 4 hours at 104º F.

PER SERVING: calories 330, protein 9g, carbohydrate 21g, fat 19g, sugar 11g
PERCENT DAILY VALUES: potassium 17%, vitamin A 112%, vitamin C 11%, calcium 12%, iron 11%, vitamin E 49%, thiamin 9%, folate 7%, vitamin K 21%, phosphorus 20%, magnesium 26%, zinc 9%, copper 23%, manganese 50%, chromium 7%, dietary fiber 25%

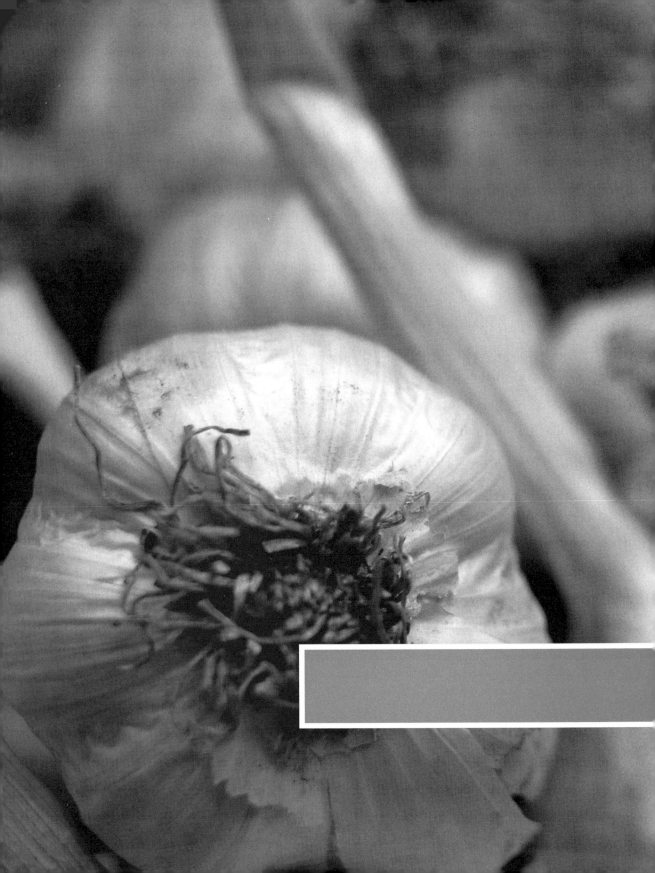

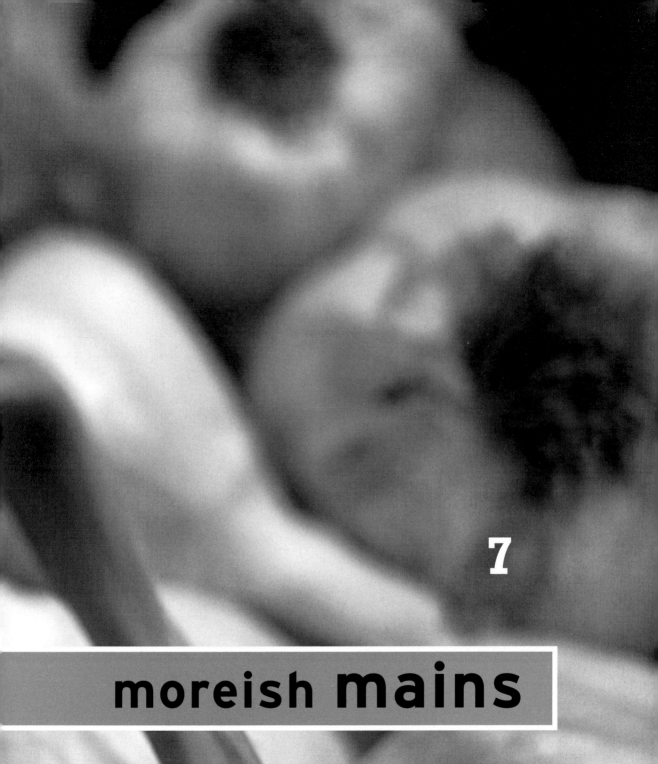

7

moreish mains

remember to breathe

WE CAN NEVER tell how healthy someone is from the outside. I know some people who work out like crazy, just so they can eat anything they want without worrying about gaining weight. Health is so much more than our weight. Exercise should not only include cardio, weight training, and stretching, but nutrition and decreasing mental stress are essential as well. Mind, body, and spirit balance is essential for total radiant health.

While we may think stress is something that only affects us in a particular moment, stress actually contributes to a sum total. We get taken down with illness when we fill up and exceed our maximum capacity. High levels of stress are known to kill. According to PhDs Lyle Miller and Alma Dell Smith, authors of *The Stress Solution*, chronic stress kills through suicide, violence, heart attack, stroke, and even cancer. People wear down to a final, fatal breakdown. Because physical and mental resources are eventually depleted, the symptoms of chronic stress are difficult to treat and may require extended medical as well as behavioral treatment and stress management. If you hate being sick, like I do, you'll want to do your best to keep stress at minimum levels. Some kinds of stress are easier to control than others:

ENVIRONMENTAL STRESSORS

Environmental stressors include the air we breathe and the toxins in our home and workplace. These include carbon monoxide, primarily from automobile exhaust; hydrocarbons like methane, ethane, propane, and butane; volatile organic compounds (VOCs) like gasoline, solvents, cleaning solutions; and nitrogen oxides that can react with hydrocarbon in the atmosphere to contribute to photochemical smog. U.S. National Pollutant Emission Estimates report that 25,393 tons of nitrogen oxide were released in the United States in 1999.

PHYSICAL STRESSORS

Physical stress comes from using our bodies when we exercise and work, and even from lack of rest and sleep. As workplaces demand longer hours, they create emotional stress that can affect us physically.

EMOTIONAL STRESSORS

Pressures of daily life, work, responsibilities, and challenges in our days create emotional stress.

NUTRITIONAL STRESSORS

Eating foods that are hard on our body, difficult for us to digest, or don't provide enough nutrients creates nutritional stress.

SOME STRESSORS CAN'T BE EASILY DECREASED

Some environmental stress, like air pollution, can't be controlled. We can decrease our exposure to them by being aware of the products we bring into our home and by keeping our home environment toxic-free. And having more green plants around creates clean air.

Physical stress can be good and bad. Exercise is good for us. But overexercising might make us sick, because we exceed the maximum sum total of stress our bodies can handle. Marathon runners, for example, who train really hard just before a race are susceptible to getting sick, because their additional physical stress pushes them over their stress threshold.

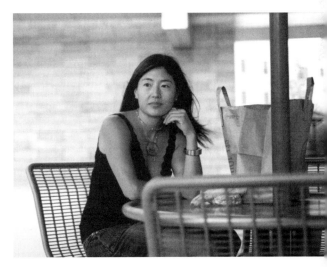

Emotional stress takes work to decrease. Taking time out of our busy day to be quiet and calm, to practice yoga, deep breathing, and meditation are all great ways to decrease stress.

Nutritional stress is the easiest to decrease. By enjoying more organic fresh whole food, we create more space in which to handle the other three types of stressors. So even if the other three stresses are high, we can handle more of them before we hit our stress threshold.

When I went 100 percent raw, within a month I'd dropped fifteen pounds. More importantly, all my allergies disappeared. And it's been over eight years since I've had a flu or cold. I used to hate being sick, and I don't miss having a stuffy nose, fever, and headaches. Because I eat so many fresh organic foods, I just don't get sick anymore. My immune system is stronger than it's ever been.

I hope to inspire you to experience vibrant health so you can get the most out of your life! By decreasing overall stress and downtime due to illness, you'll have more time to do all those things you've always wanted.

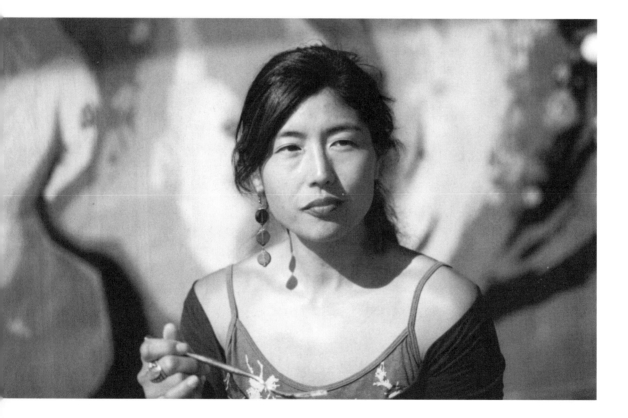

BALANCING YOUR MEALS

All my meals are nutritionally balanced. With living foods, it's important to eat enough fat to balance, ground, and keep us feeling full and satisfied.

Some folks worry about how eating fats affects their weight. Good fats are necessary for our organs and bodily functions, and they're good for our heart. The more fats we eat, the more 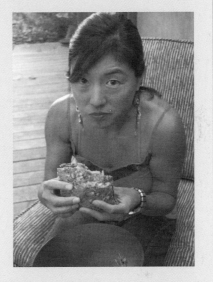 our body lets go of fats, because it knows more will be coming in. The same goes for water. The less we drink, the more our bodies retain. The more we drink, the more it lets go of.

In general, I've found balancing one-third plant fat (nuts, seeds, oils) with one-third dark leafy greens and one-third fruits works really well for me. In the summertime, though, I may bump up the fruits to about 75 percent or so, greens to about 20 percent, and just eat a handful of nuts a day. This may be too much sugar for some. I'm physically active, and the sugar fuels my body and burns right off.

I have a friend who's really thin and lean, but solid muscle. He eats at least three avocados a day and probably about a pound of nuts and seeds. I could never eat that much fat, and prefer the greens and fruits instead.

It's easy to have favorites and to fall into a pattern, but it's really important to mix up what you eat all the time. Eating a variety of nuts, seeds, fruits, and vegetables will ensure you get your full range of nutrients. Eating locally and seasonally will help mix it up.

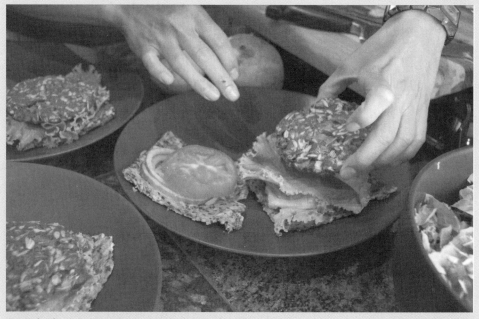

Every body is unique. So start with the 1/3, 1/3, 1/3, and adjust until you find what works for you.

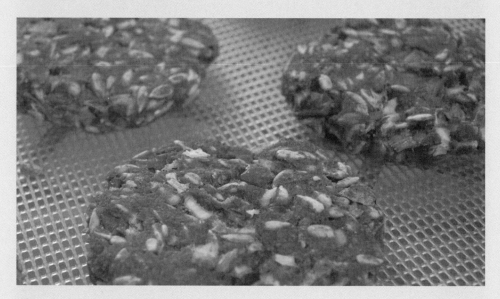

There are a couple recipes in this section where dehydration is an option. You can always opt out. If you're like me, you love your water.

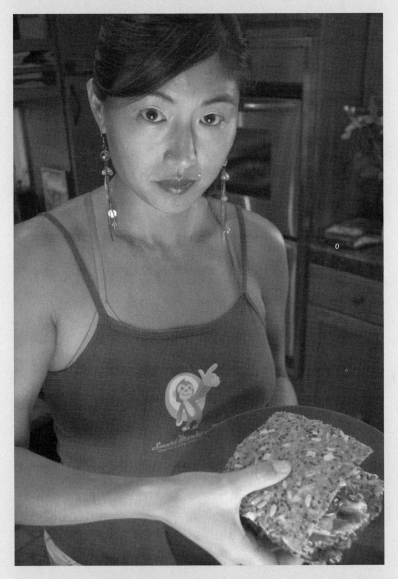

But some things like crackers or bread need to be dried to become stiff. If it's hot enough out-side with lots of sunshine, you can always dehydrate the natural energy-free way by sun-drying, too. Though not optimal, as a last resort you could always use your oven. Turn it onto the lowest setting, and let it begin to get warm. Remember, 104° F is warm to the touch. Once warm, turn off the oven. Then place your bread or item for drying in the oven until the oven cools off. Keep turning the heat back on and turn it off once it gets warm. Keep repeating until food is dry.

wrap and roll

NORI SHEETS SHOULD be labeled raw, or else they will be toasted. Nori is a sea veggie and is full of iodine, chlorophyll, and minerals from the ocean. Collard green leaves also make great wraps. They have a large surface area and lay flat, so they roll up really nice. Plus, they're packed full of chlorophyll and calcium. All good stuff!

Store leftovers in separate containers. Throw together an easy wrap as a treat the next day with leftover pâtés, cheezes, and spreads.

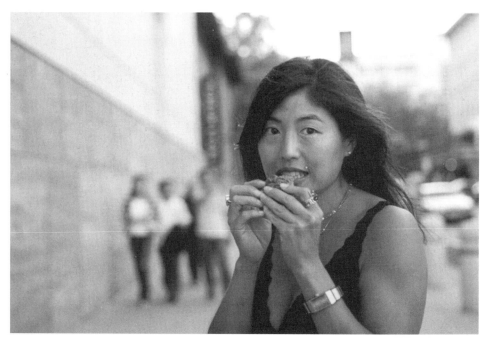

Wraps are a great handheld travel food, so you don't need dishes or cutlery to enjoy a nutritious, delicious snack on the go.

ITALIAN HERB COLLARD WRAP

MAKES 4 SERVINGS

WRAPPER

2 large collard green leaves, ribs removed and leaves halved

FILLINGS

1 batch Sunny Dill Cheeze (page 164)
2 scallions, chopped
1/2 bunch rosemary leaves, chopped
1 bunch oregano leaves, chopped
1 avocado, sliced
1/2 pint cherry tomatoes, halved
1/2 cup sun-dried tomatoes, sliced

Put about 1/3 cup of Sunny Dill Cheeze along the bottom edge of each collard green leaf. Next, layer remaining ingredients along bottom edge of each leaf.

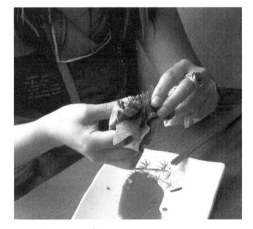

To serve, roll up each collard leaf from the bottom into a tight cylinder.

Wraps will keep for one day. Leftovers stored in separate containers will keep for two days in the fridge, so you can easily throw together a wrap as a treat the next day.

ANI'S KITCHEN TIP

Collard Wraps— De-stem and Roll

De-stem collard green leaves by cutting leaves in half and removing the hard stem. Use each half-leaf to roll up a wrap.

Before rolling, place the darker green"'top" of the leaf side down so when you roll it up it'll be on the outside and look prettier.

Spread roll fillings along the edge nearest you. Then roll up the leaf with fillings so the cut edge is on one end of the cylinder, and the natural leaf edge is on the other.

THAI SPRING ROLLS WITH DIPPING SAUCE

MAKES 4 SERVINGS

Basil, cilantro, and mint are the key herbs making this flavor authentic Thai.

THAI DIPPING SAUCE

¼ cup extra virgin olive oil
4 kaffir lime leaves
1 tablespoon Nama Shoyu
2 Thai red chilies
½ cup raw almond butter
Juice of 1 lemon, about 2 tablespoons
1 cup filtered water

FILLINGS

1 zucchini, julienned
1 cup mung bean sprouts
½ bunch basil leaves
½ bunch cilantro leaves
¼ bunch mint leaves
1 to 2 Thai chilies, finely chopped

WRAPPER

2 large collard green leaves, ribs removed, and leaves halved

To make dipping sauce, blend olive oil, lime leaves, Nama Shoyu, red chilies, almond butter, lemon juice, and water until smooth. Set aside.

To fill wrapper, lay a collard leaf flat, darker green side down, and layer filling ingredients along the bottom edge of each leaf.

To serve, roll up each collard leaf from the bottom into a tight cylinder. You can choose to make more rolls with less filling, or just four rolls with more filling. Serve with Thai Dipping Sauce.

Rolls will keep for one day. Store dipping sauce separately; it'll keep for four days in the fridge.

SAVE-THE-TUNA WRAP

MAKES 4 SERVINGS

Enjoy with Garlic Cashew Aïoli (page 127).

WRAPPER

2 large collard green leaves, ribs removed, and leaves halved

FILLINGS

1 batch Save-the-Tuna Pâté (page 166)
¼ head iceberg lettuce, shredded
1 tomato, sliced

To fill wrapper, place ¼ cup of the Save-the-Tuna Pâté along the bottom of each collard leaf half. Top with shredded lettuce and tomato.

To serve, roll up each collard leaf from the bottom into a tight cylinder.

Wrap will keep for one day. Stored separately, wrappers and filling will keep for a few days in the fridge.

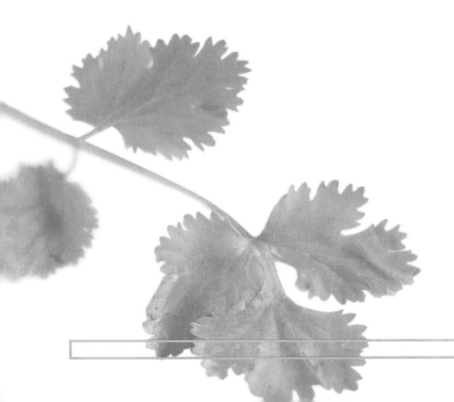

SAVE-THE-TUNA ROLL

MAKES 4 SERVINGS

FILLING

1 tablespoon wasabi powder
1 batch Save-the-Tuna Pâté (page 166)
4 romaine lettuce leaves
1 tomato, sliced
Nama Shoyu

WRAPPER

4 nori sheets

FOR DIPPING

Wasabi paste
Nama Shoyu

Mix wasabi powder with just enough water to make a thick paste. Set aside.

To fill wrapper, lay out four nori sheets. Make sure your four romaine leaves are dry, and place them along the bottom edge of each sheet of nori. Spread at least ½ cup of the Save-the-Tuna Pâté into each romaine leaf, and top with sliced tomato.

Roll up your nori almost to the top. Spread a line of wasabi with your finger along the top edge of the nori. This will help seal your roll. Roll completely.

To serve, eat whole or slice with a very sharp knife into four to six pieces. Enjoy immediately.

Serve with wasabi paste and Nama Shoyu for dipping.

Stored separately, filling will keep for a few days in the fridge.

GINGER ALMOND NORI ROLL

MAKES 4 SERVINGS

Enjoy with Japanese Miso-Shiitake Soup (page 118).

WRAPPER

4 nori sheets

FILLING

1 batch Ginger Almond Pâté (page 167)
4 cups spinach leaves
1 burdock root, also called gobo, cut lengthwise into 4 long strips
2 cups mung bean sprouts

To fill wrapper, lay out your four nori sheets. For each, spread 1 cup of dry spinach leaves on end closest to you. Top with ½ cup Ginger Almond Pâté, a quarter of the burdock root, and ½ cup mung bean sprouts.

Roll up your nori to the top and serve whole or cut into four to six pieces with a sharp knife. Serve immediately.

Stored separately, filling will keep for a few days in the fridge.

better than pastas

AS A SUBSTITUTE for cooked wheat pasta, I use my spiralizer to create long angel-hair-pasta-like strands of summer squashes. It's all about texture, and when my angel-hair noodles are tossed in marinara or pesto sauce, it feels so much like cooked angel-hair pasta. Cutting the squash in wide strips will mimic fettuccini, too. All without the heavy carbs and starches.

FETTUCCINI SQUASH NOODLES IN ALFREDO SAUCE

MAKES 4 SERVINGS

NOODLES
4 zucchini squash

SAUCE
1 batch Garlic Cashew Aïoli (page 127)
¼ teaspoon ground black pepper

To make noodles, cut the tops and bottoms off of each squash. Slice lengthwise as thinly as possible with your mandoline slicer, or a knife works fine, too. Stack and cut into wide strips, just like the shape of fettuccini pasta.

Toss noodles with Garlic Cashew Aïoli and black pepper just before serving.

OPTIONAL: Serve with Cashew Garlic Parmesan Sprinkle (page 151).

Noodles in Alfredo Sauce will keep for one day in the fridge. Store squash noodles and sauce separately to keep for a few days.

ANGEL-HAIR SQUASH PASTA IN PESTO SAUCE

MAKES 4 SERVINGS

NOODLES

> **4 zucchini squash**

SAUCE

> **1 batch Pistachio Pesto (page 150)**
> **2 cups spinach leaves**
> **2 tablespoons hemp oil**
> **Pinch sea salt**

To make noodles, cut off the tops and bottoms of each squash, and then cut in half. Use your spiralizer to spiralize the squash into angel-hair noodles.

Put noodles in a large bowl. Using the back of a spoon, mix in Pistachio Pesto or Macadamia Pesto really well. You'll notice the squash beginning to release water. This water will help mix your thick pesto with the pasta.

In a medium bowl, toss spinach with hemp oil and a pinch of salt, to taste.

To serve, place spinach leaves on bottom of four bowls or dishes. Top each with Angel-Hair Squash Pasta in Pesto Sauce.

Pasta in Pesto Sauce will keep for one day in the fridge. Store squash pasta and Pesto Sauce separately to keep for a few days.

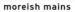

ANGEL-HAIR SQUASH NOODLES IN SUN-DRIED TOMATO MARINARA

MAKES 4 SERVINGS

This is great with Cashew Garlic Parmesan Sprinkle (page 151).

NOODLES

4 zucchini squash

SAUCE

1 batch Sun-Dried Tomato Marinara (page 126)

To make noodles, cut off the tops and bottoms of each squash, and then cut in half. Use your spiralizer to spiralize your squash into angel-hair noodles.

Toss your angel-hair noodles with marinara. Serve immediately, as it will begin to release water.

Store squash noodles and marinara separately to keep for a few days in the fridge.

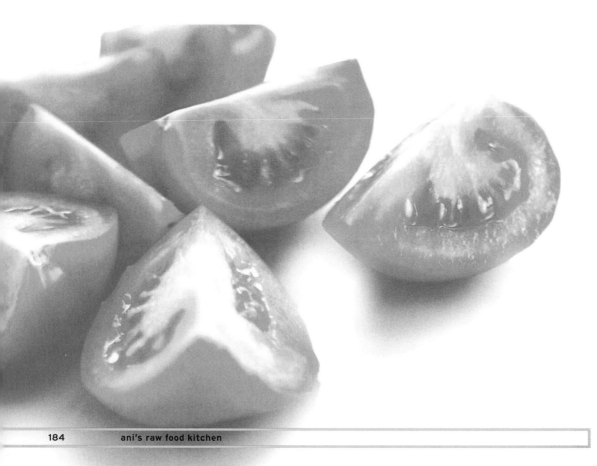

ITALIAN RAWZANIA

MAKES 4 SERVINGS

This dish uses zucchini squash thinly sliced for the pasta layers. I try to use fresh herbs whenever possible. But it's okay to use dried herbs, too. Serve with Cashew Garlic Parmesan Sprinkle (page 151).

NOODLES
3 zucchini squash

FILLINGS
½ batch Sun-Dried Tomato Marinara (page 126)
½ batch Italian Pizza Cheeze (page 161)
1 tomato, sliced
¼ cup yellow onion, sliced
½ cup black olives, pitted and chopped
½ cup sun-dried tomatoes
¼ cup oregano, fresh or dried leaves
¼ cup thyme, fresh or dried leaves

To make noodles, use a mandoline slicer or a knife to cut squash thinly into circles.

In a 8 x 9-inch baking pan (remember this makes four servings), start by layering half the squash on bottom. Top with half the Italian Pizza Cheeze, then half the tomato, half of the onion, about a ½ cup of Sun-Dried Tomato Marinara, half the olives, half the sun-dried tomatoes, oregano, and thyme.

Layer the rest of the squash. Gently push down on the zucchini layer lightly to pack. Layer remaining cheeze, tomatoes, onion, marinara, olives, sun-dried tomatoes, oregano, and thyme.

Will keep for one day in the fridge, and actually tastes better the second day once all the flavors marinate together.

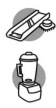

PAD THAI NOODLES
IN ALMOND KAFFIR SAUCE

MAKES 4 SERVINGS

At a glance, this recipe may seem more complex, but it's not really. Just simple noodles tossed in a yummy Pad Thai–inspired sauce with fresh Thai herbs and chilies.

Just julienne some squash, red bell pepper, and coconut meat into "noodles." If you can't find Thai baby coconuts, then substitute an extra squash instead. Look for the word "raw" on your almond butter, otherwise it'll be toasted.

NOODLES

⅓ yellow onion, thinly sliced

3 tablespoons Nama Shoyu

2 zucchini squash, green and/or yellow, julienned

1 red bell pepper, julienned

Meat from 2 Thai baby coconuts, julienned

1 cup mung bean sprouts

FRESH THAI HERBS

⅓ bunch basil chiffonade (see page 120)

⅓ bunch cilantro leaves,

⅓ bunch mint, leaves, chopped

2 Thai red chilies, seeded and chopped

ALMOND KAFFIR SAUCE

2 tablespoons minced ginger

Juice of 4 limes, about 8 tablespoons

3 tablespoons pitted dates

3 tablespoons Nama Shoyu

2 kaffir lime leaves

1 ¼ cups almond butter

¼ cup water, as needed

TOPPINGS

1 cup mung bean sprouts

⅓ cup almonds, sliced

To make noodles, marinate onion in Nama Shoyu. Set aside for at least 5 minutes to marinate and soften.

In a large bowl, combine zucchini, bell pepper, Thai baby coconut meat, and mung bean sprouts. Add marinated onions. Set aside about 2 tablespoons of the Fresh Thai Herbs and about a tablespoon of the red chilies to use as garnish just before serving. Place the rest of the herbs and chilies in with the noodles.

To make sauce, blend ginger, lime juice, Nama Shoyu, and lime leaves until smooth. Add almond butter with just enough water as needed to help blend to a thick, creamy texture.

To serve, toss noodles with sauce before serving. Place onto four plates or bowls, and top with toppings. Garnish with herbs and chili. Serve immediately.

Pad Thai will keep for one day. Store noodles, fresh herbs, and toppings separately to keep for two days. Sauce will keep for four to five days in the fridge.

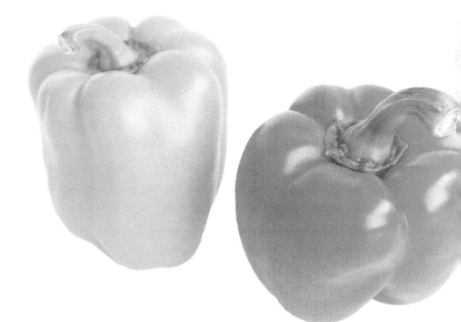

MUSHROOM RISOTTO
WITH WHITE TRUFFLE–INFUSED OLIVE OIL

MAKES 4 SERVINGS

RISOTTO

½ acorn squash, about 1 ¾ pounds, peeled and cut into 1-inch cubes

MARINATED MUSHROOMS

2 cups mushrooms, any type, sliced

3 tablespoons Nama Shoyu

KREAM

2 cloves garlic

1 teaspoon sea salt

1 ½ cups almonds

¾ cup filtered water, as needed

1 cup extra virgin olive oil

TOPPINGS

¼ cup white truffle–infused olive oil

1 scallion, chopped

To make risotto, place small batches of peeled and cubed squash into your food processor and process into small risotto-size pieces. Put in large mixing bowl and set aside.

Mix mushrooms with Nama Shoyu, and set aside to marinate and soften for at least 5 minutes.

To make kream, process garlic and salt into small pieces. Add almonds and process into a powder. Add just enough water to make a thick, creamy texture. Add olive oil last to thicken even more. Place kream in bowl with risotto and mix well. Add marinated mushrooms and mix again.

To serve, place Mushroom Risotto into four bowls. Drizzle with white truffle–infused olive oil and chopped scallion.

Will keep for three days in the fridge.

PER SERVING: calories 381, protein 14g, carbohydrate 20g, fat 31g, sugar 3g
PERCENT DAILY VALUES: potassium 36%, vitamin A 14%, vitamin C 38%, calcium 20%, iron 25%, vitamin D 9%, vitamin E 106%, thiamin 31%, riboflavin 38%, niacin 28%, folate 13%, vitamin K 52%, phosphorus 38%, magnesium 51%, zinc 13%, copper 44%, manganese 83%, dietary fiber 39%

more main dishes that make you sing

HERE ARE MORE of my favorite mains. They make me sing out loud, they're so delightful.

I hope they'll make you break into song, too. These recipes have all been inspired by cravings I've had for the cooked versions I'd stopped eating, and by requests fueled from the cravings of friends and customers.

BAJA CHEEZE BURRITO WITH TACO NUT MEAT AND RED PEPPER CORN SALSA

MAKES 4 SERVINGS

Cabbage leaves work great instead of cooked tortillas for these burritos. Just peel four full leaves off a head of cabbage. Green cabbage leaves are softer and easier to peel away whole. But red cabbage leaves look really pretty. The leaves naturally form a cup, which you can fill with taco meat, cheeze, and salsa. Hold in your hands to eat, and crunch into a deliciously fresh burrito.

TORTILLA SHELLS
4 cabbage leaves, green or red

FILLING
2 cups spinach leaves
2 tablespoons extra virgin olive oil
Pinch sea salt
1 batch Baja Cheeze (page 164)
1 batch Taco Nut Meat (page 154)
1 batch Red Pepper Corn Salsa (page 151)

Toss spinach leaves with olive oil and sea salt. Put into the bottom of each cabbage cup. Top with Baja Cheeze, Taco Nut Meat, and Red Pepper Corn Salsa.

Will keep for one day. Store cabbage shells, cheeze, salsa, and spinach separately to keep for two to three days. Taco meat will keep for four days in the fridge when stored separately.

POLENTA WITH MUSHROOM RAGOUT

MAKES 4 SERVINGS

This delicious ragout is made up of two parts. The first is a blended mush-room gravy; the second is chopped mushrooms, celery, and thyme. Mix them together and you have a beautiful ragout to enjoy over your polenta.

POLENTA

1 1/2 teaspoons sea salt
1 clove garlic
1/8 teaspoon ground black pepper
1 1/2 cups cashews, dry
2 cups corn kernels, fresh or frozen (about 1 1/2 pounds)
Juice of 1/2 lemon, about 1 tablespoon
1 1/2 tablespoons yellow onion, chopped

MUSHROOM GRAVY

1/3 cup extra virgin olive oil
3/4 cup mushrooms, any kind
1/3 cup water
1 1/2 teaspoons apple cider vinegar
1 clove garlic, minced
1/2 teaspoon sea salt

RAGOUT

2 cups mushrooms, any kind, chopped
1/2 stalk celery, chopped
2 teaspoons fresh thyme

To make polenta, process salt, garlic, and black pepper first. Then add cashews and process. Place in a bowl. Next, pulse corn kernels with lemon juice. Place into bowl with cashews and onion. Mix well. Set aside.

To make gravy, blend olive oil, 3/4 cup mushrooms, water, vinegar, garlic, and salt until smooth. Pour gravy into a bowl.

To make ragout, stir 2 cups mushrooms, celery, and thyme into the gravy base.

To serve, use an ice cream scooper to scoop polenta onto four plates. Drizzle with ragout, and serve with a sprig of fresh rosemary as garnish.

Will keep for two days in the fridge.

PER SERVING: calories 550, protein 13g, carbohydrate 29g, fat 29g, sugar 7g
PERCENT DAILY VALUES: potassium 21%, vitamin C 12%, calcium 5%, iron 27%, vitamin D 13%, vitamin E 13%, thiamin 19%, riboflavin 27%, niacin 25%, vitamin B6 19%, folate 17%, pantothenic acid 19%, vitamin K 53%, phosphorus 39%, magnesium 38%, zinc 22%, copper 72%, manganese 31%, selenium 10%, dietary fiber 16%

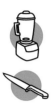

STUFFED ANAHEIM CHILIES WITH MOLE SAUCE

MAKES 4 SERVINGS

I always loved chili rellenos, but couldn't enjoy them, because they're dipped in egg and made with dairy cheese. So I was inspired to create a raw version that tastes even better!

You can choose to put these stuffed chilies in your dehydrator for 4 to 6 hours before serving. This'll marinate the cheeze full of the Anaheim flavor, while softening the chili as if it were cooked. And it's nice to serve slightly warm on a colder day.

CHILIES

4 Anaheim chili peppers
4 tablespoons extra virgin olive oil
1 batch Black-Pepper Cheeze (page 161)

MOLE SAUCE

¼ teaspoon dried chipotle
1 tablespoon pitted dates
1½ tablespoons carob powder
1 teaspoon ground cinnamon
⅓ cup extra virgin olive oil
1½ stalks celery, chopped
½ tomato, chopped
¼ teaspoon sea salt
2 tablespoons water, as needed

To make chilies, slice an opening into your peppers lengthwise. Be careful not to cut all the way through. Remove seeds. If you like it spicy, leave a few of the seeds in the peppers.

Coat inside and outside of each pepper with 1 tablespoon of olive oil. Then stuff each pepper full of Black-Pepper Cheeze.

To make Mole Sauce, blend chipotle, dates, carob powder, cinnamon, olive oil, celery, tomato, salt, and water until smooth.

To serve, place a chili pepper on each of four plates. Drizzle with Mole Sauce.

OPTIONAL: Dehydrate stuffed peppers 4 to 6 hours at 104° F until desired softness. Serve warm with Mole Sauce.

Chilies will keep for two days, and the Mole Sauce will keep for four days in the fridge when stored separately.

SAVE-THE-SALMON PATTIES WITH HOLLANDAISE SAUCE

MAKES 4 SERVINGS

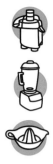

You may choose to dehydrate these patties for 5 hours before serving. This dries the outside layer and makes it look just like a real salmon cake. Plus, it's nice to serve raw foods slightly warmed on cold days.

SAVE-THE-SALMON PATTIES
Pulp from 5 peeled and juiced carrots
1 batch Sunny Dill Cheeze (page 164)
2 tablespoons yellow onion, chopped
1 teaspoon sea salt
1 tablespoon dulse flakes

HOLLANDAISE SAUCE
Juice of 3 lemons, about 6 tablespoons
1/3 cup water
2/3 cups almond
2/3 teaspoon sea salt
1/3 teaspoon turmeric
1/3 cup extra virgin olive oil

To make patties, place carrot pulp into a large bowl with Sunny Dill Cheeze. Add onion, salt, and dulse. Mix well. Divide into four balls and flatten each into a patty shape.

To make Hollandaise Sauce, blend lemon juice, water, almonds, salt, and turmeric until smooth. Add oil and blend until thick. If you need to help the Hollandaise keep moving in the blender, use a spatula to stir it up. But be careful and don't touch the blades, or it'll eat up your spatula.

Patties will keep for two days non-dehydrated and four days dehydrated. Hollandaise will keep for five days in the fridge when stored separately.

OPTIONAL: Dehydrate patties for 5 hours at 104º F. Serve warm topped with Hollandaise Sauce.

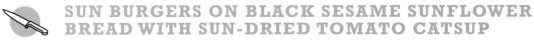

SUN BURGERS ON BLACK SESAME SUNFLOWER BREAD WITH SUN-DRIED TOMATO CATSUP

MAKES 4 SERVINGS

You may want to dehydrate your burgers for a few hours before eating. Drying makes them a bit more firm, like a burger patty, as opposed to a pâté. And you can serve them warm!

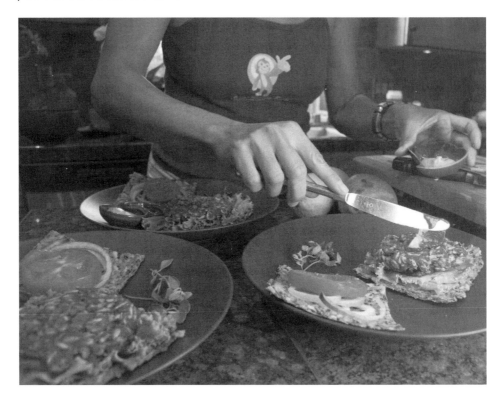

SUN BURGERS

2 stalks celery, chopped, about ¾ cup

¼ cup yellow onion, chopped

½ cup red bell peppers, chopped

1 teaspoon sea salt

2 teaspoons oregano, fresh or dried

1 cup sunflower seeds, ground

½ cup flax seeds, ground

½ cup water

8 slices of Black Sesame Sunflower Bread (page 153)

1 batch Sun-Dried Tomato Catsup (page 129)
1 batch Hot Mustard Sauce (page 130)

1 tomato, sliced
Leaves of your favorite lettuce

To make burgers, place celery, onion, bell peppers, salt, oregano, sunflower seeds, and flax seeds in a bowl, adding water last. Mix well. Form four balls and flatten into burger patties.

To serve, enjoy between slices of Black Sesame Sunflower Bread with Sun-Dried Tomato Catsup and Hot Mustard Sauce, topped with slices of tomatoes and lettuce.

Will keep for one day. Non-dehydrated burgers will keep for two days, and dehydrated burgers will keep for four days when stored separately. Store bread, catsup, and mustard separately to keep for five days. Store toppings separately to keep for two days in the fridge.

OPTIONAL: Dehydrate burgers for three hours at 104° F, serve warm.

MARINATED PORTABELLO STEAK AND BRAZIL-BROCCOLI MASH WITH MUSHROOM GRAVY

MAKES 4 SERVINGS

STEAK

4 portabello mushrooms, stems removed
¼ cup extra virgin olive oil
⅓ cup Nama Shoyu
1 tablespoon finely chopped rosemary

MASH

1 batch Brazil-Broccoli Mash (page 143)

GRAVY

1 batch Mushroom Gravy (page 190)

4 sprigs rosemary

To make steaks, in a large bowl, coat mushrooms in oil, Nama Shoyu, and rosemary. Set aside for an hour or two to marinate and soften.

To serve, slice each mushroom into 4 to 5 thick strips and serve on top of a scoop of Brazil-Broccoli Mash. Drizzle with Mushroom Gravy, garnish with a sprig of rosemary before serving.

Will keep for one day. Store portabello steaks separately to keep for two days. Mash and gravy will keep for several days in the fridge when stored separately.

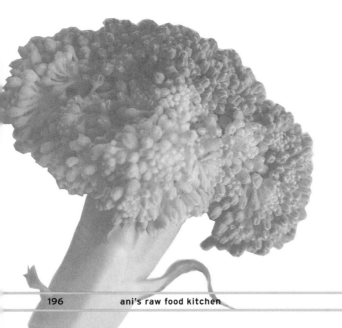

PIZZA WITH SUN-DRIED TOMATOES, BLACK OLIVES, AND FRESH ITALIAN HERBS

MAKES 4 SERVINGS

PIZZA

4 slices of Black Sesame Sunflower Bread (page 153)
½ batch Italian Pizza Cheeze (page 161)
½ batch Sun-Dried Tomato Marinara (page 126)

TOPPINGS

1 tomato, sliced
¼ cup black olives, pitted and chopped
¼ cup sun-dried tomatoes, sliced
1 tablespoon fresh oregano
¼ cup fresh basil, torn
4 teaspoons extra virgin olive oil

To make pizza, top each slice of Black Sesame Sunflower Bread with a layer of Italian Pizza Cheeze and Sun-Dried Tomato Marinara.

Top your pizza with slices of tomato, olives, sun-dried tomatoes, oregano, and basil. Drizzle with olive oil before serving.

Will keep for one day in the fridge. Store bread, cheeze, and marinara separately to keep for four days. Keep toppings stored separately to keep for a couple days. It's a great way to have all the pieces to easily throw together pizzas.

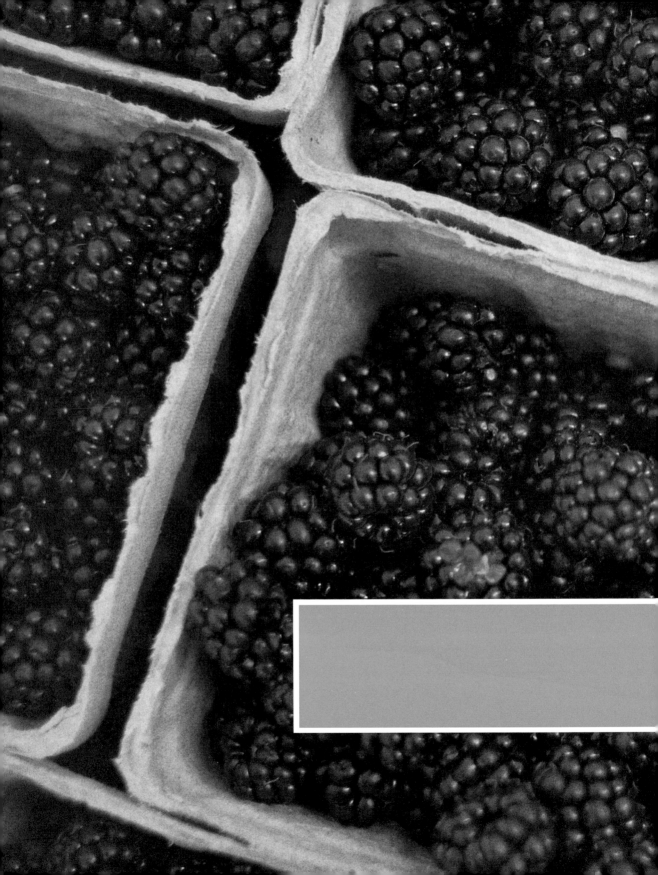

8

decadent
desserts

beauty is more than skin deep

BEAUTY ISN'T JUST on the surface. It radiates from feeling great and being happy. The right nutrients from whole organic fresh foods can make you glow from the inside out.

Many beauty products have synthetic chemical ingredients added. These cocktails of toxins have been found to cause cancer and reproductive damage over years of sustained use. Our skin is our largest organ and absorbs everything we put on it, just like we're drinking it into our mouths. So I'm sure to use only natural edible moisturizers on my hair and skin.

People comment on my skin often. I think it's from the glow that living foods give everyone who eats this way. Besides eating and drinking a lot of water, here are some of the beautifiers I use.

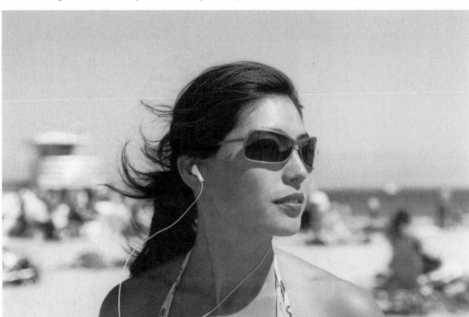

COCONUT OIL

I love using coconut oil from my kitchen to moisturize my whole body. It feels and smells great. If you don't want to smell like a piña colada, you can buy oils with less or no scent. These are usually the lower-cost edible organic oils, too.

I also love putting coconut oil on the ends of my hair. It's known to improve hair quality. In southern India, women apply coconut oil to their hair every day for long, lustrous locks.

Coconut is also known to improve complexion. It gives your skin a beautiful moisturized finish.

ALOE

For scrapes, burns, scars, or rashes, try squeezing aloe gel from a freshly picked leaf. You'll be amazed by the rapid pain relief and how fast you'll heal. Plus, it helps prevent scarring.

For sunburns, mash up ripe strawberries and apply directly to burned skin for 5 to 10 minutes. Or place peeled, thinly sliced cucumbers on burned skin and remove when cucumbers get warm. Cucumbers are also good for delicate skin areas like our neck or eyes. And when placed on our eyes for 20 minutes, sliced cucumbers reduce puffiness and relieve tired eyes.

HEMP

Hemp needs no pesticides or fertilizers to grow. It's low maintenance and grows just about anywhere. It's an ideal crop for organic sustainable farming.

Perfectly balanced with omega 3 and omega 6, it's also great for sustainable human health. With its full amino acid spectrum, it provides a complete protein and is high in trace mineral content.

I use hemp seed oil to nourish my skin and hair on a cellular level. It's easily absorbed into my skin, and the omegas go straight to work for me. Just apply it directly onto the palms of your hands and then work into your hair or skin.

SUN PROTECTION

A diet rich in EFAs (essential fatty acids) from hemp, flax, and walnuts helps our skin in its natural protection against the sun. Eating antioxidant-rich foods kills free radicals and helps shield our skin from sun damage. So it's possible to actually eat your sunblock—by enjoying more fresh organic whole foods. And remember to wear your sunglasses.

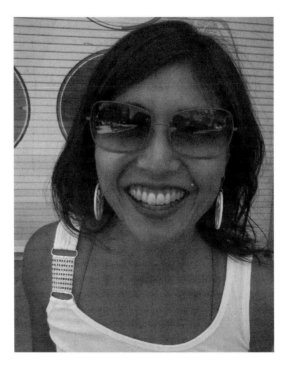

beauty products i can live without

NAIL POLISH

My dad never let me wear nail polish growing up. I'd sneak it on at school and take it off before going back home at the end of the day. I can't believe it took me so long to understand why nail polish is unhealthy, especially when it smells so awful.

Colored nails may look pretty, but polish contains toxic chemicals like dibutyl phthalate (DBP), toluene, and formaldehyde. In 2004 the European Union banned the use of DBP from cosmetics, citing a link to reproductive harm. Yet it's still used here in the United States. You can smell these toxic chemicals. And they enter our body through our lungs and are absorbed through our nails. Toxins in most nail polishes are poisonous to our reproductive system and are known carcinogens, as reported by the Organic Consumers Association.

I like bare nails myself and use a buffer to shine them without relying on chemicals.

ANTIBACTERIAL SOAP

There's both *good* and *bad* bacteria. Decreasing bad bacteria prevents illness, but antibacterial soaps kill both the good and the bad strains. To strengthen our immune system, it's important for us to be exposed to everyday germs so our bodies can practice combating them. Plus, the use of antibacterial products is causing stronger strains of superbugs to emerge.

Most antibacterial soaps use the chemical triclosan, which is used, just like pesticide, to kill bacteria. This chemical is toxic to your liver and kidneys. And when exposed to UV light, it reacts to create cancer, reproductive and developmental problems, and immune system damage.

Try using tea tree oil instead of chemical antibacterial products. It kills fungus and bacteria, including those resistant to some antibiotics. Tea tree oil can be used topically as an antiseptic; it also can be used as an anti-infective for bacterial infections, acne, and fungal infections like athlete's foot. I also use it on insect bites and other minor skin irritations.

I got to swim in a tea tree lake outside Byron Bay in Australia. The water was tea color from the tea tree leaves that fell in it off surrounding trees. It was amazing; my hair and skin were soft for a week!

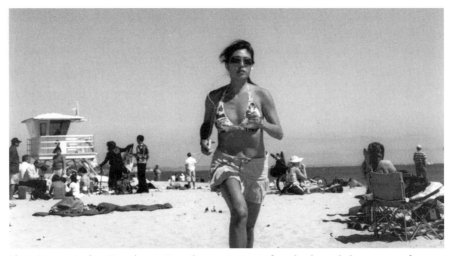

I love to sweat when I work out. It pushes toxins out of my body and cleanses me from the inside out. Sweat works to cool my body and regulates my temperature.

ANTIPERSPIRANT

I don't use antiperspirants or deodorants, because they clog pores with aluminum to block sweat, and they also contain the chemical preservative paraben. Aluminum has been linked to the development of Alzheimer's disease, and paraben has been linked to breast cancer.

You'll notice as you increase the amount of fresh organics in your diet, your body odor will diminish. As your insides cleanse and become cleaner, your sweat won't smell as strong.

FRAGRANCES

Ninety-five percent of chemicals used in fragrances are synthetic chemicals that come from petroleum. They include benzene derivatives, aldehydes, and many other known toxins capable of causing cancer, birth defects, central nervous system disorders, and allergic reactions.

If you like scents, try essential oils. Essential oils are the pure "essence" of a plant and have been found to provide psychological and physical benefits. The aroma of natural essential oil stimulates the brain to trigger a reaction, and naturally occurring chemicals are taken into the lungs, providing physical benefits. They even work as a natural repellent and pesticide. Use citronella oil in summertime to keep mosquitoes away.

FIGHT FLAB

I lost 15 pounds during my first month of eating only fresh whole organic living foods. Believe me when I say I was stuffing myself on delicious foods every day. It's not really a surprise when I think of all the water and fiber I was filling up on. And the water and fiber were washing and sweeping all my cells clean. I was letting go of stored toxins and fat; my fat cells were shrinking. Plus, living foods put tone back into my skin and muscles. Just like facial products that put vitamins and antioxidants in to tone skin, I'm eating these same nutrients.

Losing body fat, exercising, strength training, and natural living can make positive changes to your overall health and well-being.

Enjoy live-food desserts without guilt or worry! By eating the live-food desserts in this section, you might actually *lose* weight! Even more important, you'll feel better and your body will thank you for it.

I loved eating baked goods of all types: cookies, cakes, croissants, scones, and more. When I discovered organic living cuisine, I was thrilled even the desserts were 100 percent guilt-free.

Living-cuisine desserts are not only good for the planet since they're cruelty free, but they're good for our health as well. They're naturally sweetened with fruit and fiber, instead of refined white sugar. And my recipes use protein- and calcium-rich nuts and seeds, rather than bleached white flour.

Live desserts are nutrient dense. Every bite gives our body healthy vitamins, minerals, antioxidants, and phytonutrients that strengthen our immune system, defend against bacteria and viruses, reduce inflammation, and prevent cancer and heart disease.

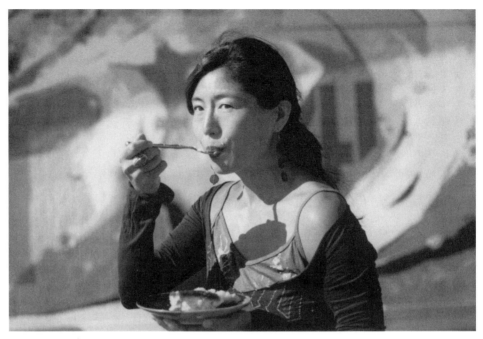

If I had to choose my favorite recipes, they'd be found in this desserts chapter. My insatiable sweet tooth and background as a pastry chef means desserts are my favorite meal.

When we developed the brownies for SmartMonkey Foods, they were about half the size of a baked brownie but cost twice as much. Potential customers often question the high cost. Our brownie is nutrient dense; while I *could* add a cup of flour and a cup of sugar (two of the cheapest ingredients around) to add bulk, the sugar and flour aren't essential (or healthy) ingredients. They only add stress on the body.

Flour and water can be mixed together to make paste to use for papier-mâché, as well as to hang concert posters around town. Imagine how hard our digestive system needs to work to break down a sticky paste when we eat it. This places strain and stress on our body, using up energy rather than revitalizing us. Eating anything fresh and raw—whether it's a yummy soup or delicious dessert—is fueling our bodies. We can choose to use low-grade or high-grade fuel. I'll take some rocket fuel, thank you!

These decadent recipes all have nutrient information, so you can see how many nutrients each provides. Eat them as a meal for breakfast or any time. You *can* have your cake and eat it, too—this stuff's good for you!!

dessert soups

THESE SOUPS ARE sweet and beautiful in color, especially contrasted against the lighter kream color. Swirled together, they make a lovely ending to any meal.

STRAWBERRY KREAM SWIRL

MAKES 4 SERVINGS

SOUP

> 4 cups strawberries
> 1 cup Medjool pitted dates, or ½ cup honey, agave, or maple syrup

KREAM

> 2 cups almonds
> 1 cup water
> 4 spearmint leaves, for garnish
> 4 slices strawberry, for garnish

Puree strawberries and dates in a food processor. Pour into a mixing bowl and set aside.

To make kream, place almonds and water in blender and whip into a smooth kream. Fold kream into bowl with soup. Mix barely enough to swirl the red with the white.

To serve, scoop swirled soup and kream into four bowls.

Top each with a spearmint leaf or strawberry slice as garnish.

Will keep for two to three days in the fridge.

> **PER SERVING:** calories 273, protein 7g, carbohydrate 28g, fat 16g, sugar 18g
> **PERCENT DAILY VALUES:** potassium 28%, vitamin C 141%, calcium 20%, iron 21%, vitamin E 86%, thiamin 14%, riboflavin 35%, niacin 18%, vitamin B6 11%, folate 15%, vitamin K 5%, phosphorus 37%, magnesium 54%, zinc 17%, copper 44%, manganese 116%, selenium 5%, dietary fiber 56%

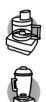

BLUEBERRY SOUP WITH CASHEW KREAM

MAKES 4 SERVINGS

SOUP
4 cups blueberries
1 cup Medjool pitted dates or ½ cup honey, agave, or maple syrup

CASHEW KREAM
2 cups cashews
1 cup water
1 batch Puckering Lemon Mint Ice (page 230)

Puree blueberries and dates in a food processor. Scoop into a bowl and set aside.

To make Cashew Kream, blend cashews and water into a smooth kream. Fold into soup. Mix slightly to swirl blue and white. Scoop puree into four bowls.

Top with Lemon Ice.

Will keep for two to three days in the fridge.

PER SERVING: calories 250, protein 7g, carbohydrate 30g, fat 15g, sugar 21g
PERCENT DAILY VALUES: potassium 23%, vitamin A 2%, vitamin C 24%, calcium 6%, iron 28%, vitamin E 9%, thiamin 14%, riboflavin 13%, niacin 11%, vitamin B6 16%, folate 16%, vitamin K 66%, phosphorus 38%, magnesium 52%, zinc 28%, copper 85%, manganese 58%, selenium 14%, dietary fiber 36%

FUZZY NAVEL CON KREAM

MAKES 4 SERVINGS

3 oranges, peeled and seeded

1 cup Medjool pitted dates, or ¼ cup honey, agave, or maple syrup

1 vanilla bean

Water, as needed

1 batch Cashew Kream (page 208)

Blend oranges, dates, vanilla bean, and water until smooth. Pour puree into four bowls.

To serve, scoop Cashew Kream on top of each bowl of soup.

Will keep for two to three days in the fridge.

PER SERVING: calories 282, protein 6g, carbohydrate 33g, fat 16g, sugar 20g

PERCENT DAILY VALUES: potassium 24%, vitamin C 87%, calcium 9%, iron 26%, vitamin E 3%, thiamin 16%, riboflavin 12%, niacin 9%, vitamin B6 15%, folate 21%, vitamin K 31%, phosphorus 38%, magnesium 52%, zinc 27%, copper 83%, manganese 35%, selenium 14%, dietary fiber 32%

pies and cobblers

IT MAY BE hard to imagine a raw, uncooked, delicious pie or cobbler. But you'll soon be a believer. Try serving without a mention of it being raw, and you'll see folks won't notice anything other than it tastes amazing. And it's good for you!

Pies are sliced and served on a crust, while the crust of a cobbler crumbles and mixes with the filling. Both are equally tasty, just different in texture and presentation.

Pies and cobbler recipes make one pie. These will keep for two to three days in your fridge.

ALL-AMERICAN APPLE PIE

MAKES ONE PIE

Have fun choosing whichever types of apples you'd like for the filling. The flavor of your raw pie will be determined by the flavor of the apples you use.

ALMOND PIE CRUST

2 cups almonds, dry
1 teaspoon sea salt
2 cups pitted dates

SYRUP

½ cup pitted dates
1 orange, peeled and seeded
Splash of water, as needed

FILLING

5 cups apples, peeled, seeded, thinly sliced, about 5 or 6 apples
1 cup raisins
2 tablespoons ground cinnamon

To make crust, pulse almonds and salt in food processor until nuts are in small pieces. You want your crust to have chunks of almonds in it, so don't overprocess. Use some of the finer powder to "flour" the bottom of your pie dish.

Slowly add dates into processor in small batches to mix with almond bits. The dates will bind the almonds to form a dough. Press dough into the bottom of "floured" pie pan. Set aside.

To make syrup, place orange into your blender first. Then add dates and blend. If needed, add small amounts of water to help everything mix well. Set aside.

To make filling, place sliced apples in a large bowl with raisins. Toss with cinnamon and syrup. Spoon filling into pie crust.

Will keep for two days in the fridge.

FOR 16 SERVINGS, PER SERVING: calories 230, protein 5g, carbohydrates 39g, fat 8g, sugar 21g
PERCENT DAILY VALUES: potassium 13%, vitamin C 13%, calcium 8%, iron 9%, vitamin E 23%, thiamin 6%, riboflavin 11%, niacin 6%, vitamin B6 6%, folate 4%, vitamin K 3%, phosphorus 11%, magnesium 16%, zinc 5%, copper 15%, manganese 34%, chromium 5%, dietary fiber 26%

PECAN CHAI PIE ON CASHEW CRUST

MAKES ONE PIE

CASHEW CRUST

1 cup cashews, dry

1 vanilla bean, scraped

1 teaspoon sea salt

1 ½ cup pitted dates (Medjool, khadrawhi, or other semi-soft date)

1 ½ cups shredded coconut

SYRUP

1 medium orange, zested, peeled, and seeded

1 cup pitted dates

1 tablespoon ground cinnamon

1 ¼ teaspoon ground cardamom

1 teaspoon grated nutmeg

Splash of water, as needed

FILLING

4 cups pecans, dry

To make crust, pulse cashews, vanilla, and salt in your food processor. Slowly add dates and process into a dough-like consistency. Empty into a bowl.

Use some of the shredded coconut to "flour" the bottom of a pie pan. Mix remaining coconut into the bowl with the cashew mixture. Press into "floured" pie pan.

To make syrup, place orange pulp into the bottom of a blender. Add dates, cinnamon, cardamom, and nutmeg and blend. Add a splash of water as needed to make a thick syrup. Set aside.

To make filling, mix pecans, syrup, and 1 tablespoon orange zest well. Spoon filling into pie crust.

Will keep for four to five days in the fridge.

FOR 16 SERVINGS, PER SERVING: calories 300, protein 5g, carbohydrates 25g, fat 21g, sugar 16g
PERCENT DAILY VALUES: potassium 11%, vitamin C 9%, calcium 4%, iron 10%, vitamin E 6%, thiamin 15%, riboflavin 4%, niacin 4%, vitamin B6 7%, folate 5%, vitamin K 6%, phosphorus 14%, magnesium 18%, zinc 13%, copper 31%, manganese 80%, selenium 5%, dietary fiber 25%

PERSIMMON PIE

MAKES ONE PIE

CASHEW CRUST
1 batch crust, from Pecan Chai Pie recipe (page 212)

SYRUP
1 cup pitted dates
1 tablespoon ground cinnamon
1 cup water, as needed

FILLING
4 cups ripe persimmons, peeled and sliced (about 7 to 8 persimmons)

To prepare crust, first use some of the shredded coconut to "flour" the bottom of a pie pan. Press crust into "floured" pie pan.

To make syrup, blend dates, cinnamon, and water until mixed well.

To make filling, mix persimmon slices with syrup. Spoon into pie crust.

Will keep for two days in the fridge.

FOR 16 SERVINGS, PER SERVING: calories 170, protein 3g, carbohydrates 24g, fat 5g, sugar 14g
PERCENT DAILY VALUES: potassium 8%, vitamin A 5%, vitamin C 14%, calcium 2%, iron 8%, thiamin 2%, riboflavin 2%, niacin 3%, vitamin B6 4%, folate 3%, vitamin K 5%, phosphorus 7%, magnesium 9%, zinc 4%, copper 14%, manganese 16%, selenium 4%, dietary fiber 14%

SUMMER BERRY COBBLER

MAKES ONE COBBLER

Our bodies need antioxidants to protect us from diseases like cancer and heart disease. Berries offer the highest levels of super-healthy antioxidants, and just one cup provides all the disease-fighting antioxidants you need in a single day. So eat up!

CRUST

    1 cup pumpkin seeds, dry
    1 cup almonds, dry
    3/4 teaspoon sea salt
    4 tablespoons extra virgin olive oil
    1/2 cup pitted dates

SYRUP

    1 cup blueberries
    1/2 cup pitted dates
    1/4 cup water, as needed

TOPPING

    1 1/2 cup blackberries and/or blueberries

To make crust, pulse pumpkin seeds, almonds, salt, and olive oil in food processor until mixture becomes a dough-like consistency. Slowly add dates and mix into a "dough." Cover the bottom of a small pie dish with the cobbler crust.

To make syrup, blend 1 cup blueberries and and 1/2 cup dates, adding enough water as needed to blend into a thick, syrupy texture.

To serve, pour the berry syrup on top of the crust. Top with 1 1/2 cups of berries.

Will keep for two days in the fridge.

FOR 16 SERVINGS, PER SERVING: calories 215, protein 7g, carbohydrates 18g, fat 12g, sugar 11g
PERCENT DAILY VALUES: potassium 9%, vitamin C 4%, calcium 4%, iron 15%, vitamin E 15%, thiamin 4%, riboflavin 8%, niacin 4%, vitamin B6 3%, folate 4%, vitamin K 17%, phosphorus 22%, magnesium 27%, zinc 10%, copper 17%, manganese 39%, selenium 2%, dietary fiber 14%

FRESH MANGO COBBLER

MAKES ONE COBBLER

This cobbler will blow your mind. It's so yummy! Make sure to choose perfectly ripe mangoes, the type without fibers if possible. The flavor of your mangoes will fully determine the flavor of your cobbler.

CRUST

> 3 cups pecans, dry
> 1 vanilla bean, scraped
> ¾ teaspoon sea salt
> ¾ cup pitted dates

SYRUP

> ¾ cup pitted dates
> 3 tablespoons coconut oil
> ½ vanilla bean
> ⅔ cup water, as needed

FILLING

> 3 to 4 ripe mangoes, peeled, seeded, sliced, about 6 cups

To make crust, process pecans, vanilla bean, and salt into a powder in your food processor. Add ¾ cup pitted dates and process until mixed well. Sprinkle half of the crust onto bottom of pie dish, and set aside. Don't bother rinsing out your food processor after making the crust; the leftover crumbs will add in with the syrup ingredients.

To make syrup, process ¾ cup dates, oil, vanilla bean, and water as needed to make a thick syrup. Set aside.

To make filling, place sliced mango into a large mixing bowl. Toss with the syrup. Spoon onto cobbler crust.

To serve, top with remaining half of the crust.

Will keep for two days in the fridge.

FOR 16 SERVINGS, PER SERVING: calories 233, protein 3g, carbohydrates 22g, fat 16g, sugar 16g
PERCENT DAILY VALUES: potassium 8%, vitamin A 7%, vitamin C 20%, calcium 3%, iron 4%, vitamin E 7%, thiamin 11%, riboflavin 4%, niacin 4%, vitamin B6 7%, folate 4%, pantothenic acid 4%, vitamin K 4%, phosphorus 7%, magnesium 9%, zinc 9%, copper 17%, manganese 48%, selenium 2%, dietary fiber 16%

FRESH MISSION FIG AND PEAR TART

MAKES ONE TART

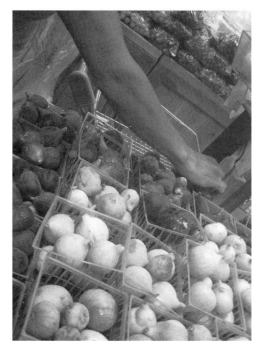

CRUST

    3 cups cashews, dry
    3/4 teaspoon sea salt
    1 vanilla bean, scraped
    1/2 cup pitted dates
    1/2 cup shredded coconut

TOPPING

    2 pears, cored, and sliced
    1 pint fresh figs, sliced
    1 orange, seeded and peeled
    1/2 cup pitted dates
    1 tablespoon coconut oil
    1 vanilla bean

To make crust, process cashews, salt, and vanilla bean into a powder in your food processor. Slowly add 1/2 cup dates. Process until it becomes dough-like. Place into a large bowl.

Use some of the coconut to "flour" the bottom of your tart dish. Mix the remaining coconut with crust. Press crust into the bottom of your tart dish.

To make topping, place pear and fig slices in a large bowl. Set aside. Blend orange, 1/2 cup dates, coconut oil, and vanilla bean until smooth, and pour over sliced pears and figs. Mix well.

To serve, scoop mixture onto tart crust.

Will keep for two days in the fridge.

FOR 16 SERVINGS, PER SERVING: calories 231, protein 5g, carbohydrates 24g, fat 11g, sugar 13g
PERCENT DAILY VALUES: potassium 9%, vitamin C 10%, calcium 3%, iron 10%, vitamin E 3%, thiamin 6%, riboflavin 5%, niacin 3%, vitamin B6 6%, folate 7%, pantothenic acid 5%, vitamin K 14%, phosphorus 14%, magnesium 20%, zinc 10%, copper 32%, manganese 16%, selenium 5%, dietary fiber 15%

COCONUT KREAM PIE WITH CAROB FUDGE ON BROWNIE CRUST

This recipe calls for our SmartMonkey Bars in our Carob Brownie flavor. You can also substitute with the Almond Pie Crust (page 211) or the Carob Crunch Torte (page 226).

CRUST

> 1/4 cup shredded coconut
>
> 8 SmartMonkey Bars, Carob Brownie flavor, or 1 batch Almond Pie Crust (page 211), or 1 batch Carob Crunch Torte (page 226)

SYRUP

> 1 cup pitted dates
>
> 1/2 cup carob powder
>
> 1/4 cup extra virgin olive oil
>
> 2 to 4 tablespoons water

KREAM

> Meat from 3 Thai baby coconuts, about 3 cups
>
> 1/2 cup pitted dates
>
> 1 cup filtered water, as needed

To make crust, "flour" pie dish with shredded coconut. Press bars or crust into pie dish. Set aside.

To make syrup, blend 1 cup dates, carob, olive oil, and water until smooth. Try to use as little water as possible for a thick fudge-like texture. Spread half of syrup onto pie crust. Set the other half aside to use as topping.

To make kream, place coconut meat in your blender with dates and blend. Gradually add just enough water to make a smooth coconut kream. Scoop into pie crust.

To serve, drizzle remaining syrup on top of pie.

OPTIONAL: You can substitute a batch of Cashew Coconut Pudding (page 73) for the kream filling, especially if Thai baby coconuts aren't available.

Will keep for three to four days in the fridge.

FOR 16 SERVINGS, PER SERVING: calories 330, protein 6g, carbohydrates 30g, fat 19g, sugar 21g
PERCENT DAILY VALUES: potassium 13%, vitamin C 1%, calcium 7%, iron 10%, vitamin E 27%, thiamin 3%, riboflavin 11%, niacin 7%, vitamin B6 5%, folate 5%, pantothenic acid 3%, vitamin K 6%, phosphorus 13%, magnesium 18%, zinc 6%, copper 19%, manganese 40%, selenium 5%, dietary fiber 32%

AUTUMN PUMPKIN PIE

This is the best pumpkin pie recipe in the world. It tastes even better than the pumpkin pie filling in cooked pies. Put it to the test, and it'll be gobbled up in no time, you'll see.

CRUST

¼ cup sunflower seeds
1 ¾ cup pumpkin seeds
½ teaspoon sea salt
1 cup pitted dates

SYRUP

1 cup pitted dates
1 ¼ cup water

FILLING

4 cups pumpkin, peeled, seeded, cut into 1-inch cubes (about 1 ½ pounds whole, before peeled)
2 teaspoons ground cinnamon
1 tablespoon psyllium powder

To make crust, process sunflower seeds into a fine powder in your food processor. Use this to "flour" the bottom of your pie dish.

Next, process pumpkin seeds and salt into a coarse meal. Slowly add 1 cup dates to make your dough. Press into pie dish. Set aside.

To make syrup, blend 1 cup dates with water until smooth. Set aside.

To make filling, process small batches of cubed pumpkin and cinnamon into a puree. Slowly add in the syrup. Process until completely smooth. Place pumpkin filling in a bowl and hand mix in psyllium powder really well.

To serve, scoop filling into pie crust.

Will keep for four days in the fridge.

FOR 16 SERVINGS, PER SERVING: calories 165, protein 5g, carbohydrates 21g, fat 7g, sugar 13g
PERCENT DAILY VALUES: potassium 11%, vitamin A 44%, vitamin C 5%, calcium 3%, iron 17%, vitamin E 8%, thiamin 7%, riboflavin 6%, niacin 4%, vitamin B6 5%, folate 6%, pantothenic acid 4%, vitamin K 11%, phosphorus 22%, magnesium 26%, zinc 9%, copper 17%, manganese 32%, selenium 4%, dietary fiber 14%

cakes

CAKES ARE SUPER nutrient dense, and decadently rich. I like to shape my cake by lining a container with parchment paper, then I press the cake into the container. It's easy to flip over and pull out. Peel away the parchment, frost, and enjoy. You can always just pat the cake into your favorite shape with your hands, too. If you don't have parchment paper, you can also use plastic wrap instead. Please make sure to reuse it to store your cake later.

These recipes will make one cake. Most cakes will keep for about a week in the fridge.

DEEP FOREST CAROB CAKE
WITH FUDGE FROSTING

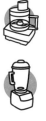

CAKE

3 ½ cup Brazil nuts
1 teaspoon sea salt
3 cups pitted dates
1 cup carob powder
3 cups shredded coconut

FROSTING

1 cup pitted dates
¼ cup carob powder
¼ cup extra virgin olive oil
1 cup water, as needed

To make cake, process Brazil nuts and salt into a powder in your food processor. Slowly add dates. Empty into a large mixing bowl and add carob and coconut. Mix well. Form into a cake shape.

To make frosting, place all ingredients into your blender. Blend into a smooth frosting. Frost your cake.

Will keep for seven days in the fridge.

FOR 24 SERVINGS, PER SERVING: calories 290, protein 5g, carbohydrates 29g, fat 6g, sugar 21g
PERCENT DAILY VALUES: potassium 12%, vitamin C 1%, calcium 7%, iron 7%, vitamin E 10%, thiamin 10%, riboflavin 3%, niacin 3%, vitamin B6 5%, folate 4%, pantothenic acid 3%, vitamin K 3%, phosphorus 18%, magnesium 24%, zinc 7%, copper 25%, manganese 24%, selenium 562%, dietary fiber 28%

COCONUT SNOW CAKE

MAKES ONE CAKE

CAKE

1 cup almonds, dry
1 cup pecans, dry
5 dehydrated bananas, chopped
3 cups pitted dates
1 vanilla bean, scraped

ICING

2 cups Medjool dates, or another soft date
1 cup pine nuts
1 vanilla bean, scraped
1 ½ cups water, as needed
½ cup shredded coconut

To make cake, finely chop almonds and pecans in food processor. Slowly add bananas, 3 cups dates, and vanilla bean and process until dough is smooth. Mold dough into desired cake shape.

To make frosting, process 2 cups dates, pine nuts, and vanilla in food processor until smooth and creamy. Add water for consistency, as needed.

To serve, spread icing on cake. Press shredded coconut into top and sides of cake.

Will keep for seven days in the fridge.

FOR 16 SERVINGS, PER SERVING: calories 375, protein 6g, carbohydrates 37g, fat 16g, sugar 28g
PERCENT DAILY VALUES: potassium 17%, vitamin C 2%, calcium 6%, iron 10%, vitamin E 18%, thiamin 8%, riboflavin 8%, niacin 8%, vitamin B6 8%, folate 5%, pantothenic acid 5%, vitamin K 8%, phosphorus 16%, magnesium 22%, zinc 10%, copper 23%, manganese 83%, selenium 4%, dietary fiber 31%

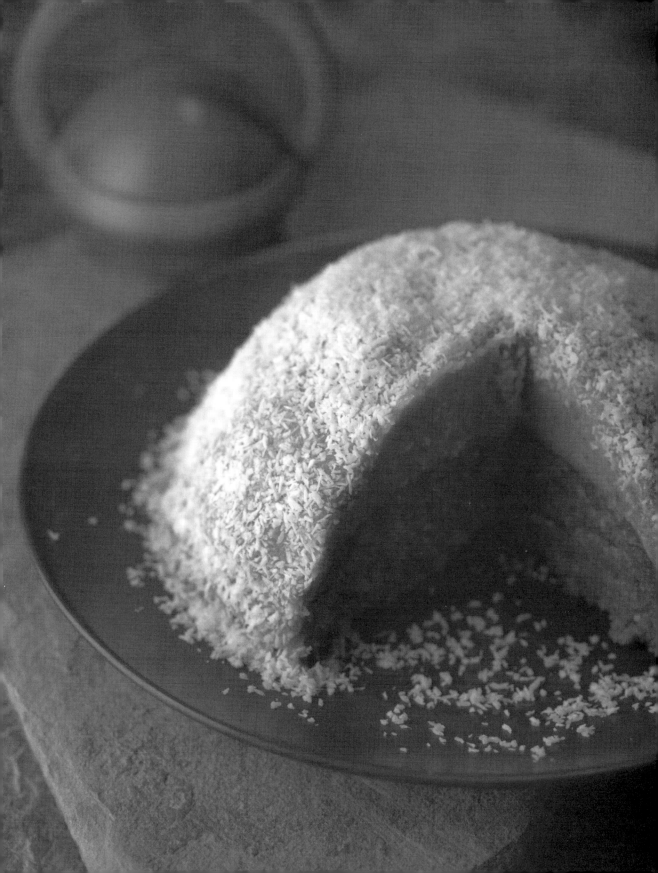

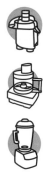

CARROT CAKE
WITH KREAM CHEEZE FROSTING

MAKES ONE CAKE

You'll notice I use agave or honey in this frosting recipe to keep the frosting whiter in color. Feel free to use 2 tablespoons pitted dates instead if you don't mind tan frosting. You'll need to use a little more water to help everything blend.

CAKE

> 5 cups carrot pulp, from about 3 pounds of juiced carrots
> 1 3/4 cups sunflower seeds
> 2 1/4 cups pitted dates
> 2 3/4 cups shredded coconut
> 1 1/2 teaspoons grated nutmeg
> 3 teaspoons ground cinnamon

KREAM CHEEZE FROSTING

> 1 1/2 cups cashews
> Juice of 1 lemon, about 2 tablespoons
> 2 tablespoons agave syrup or honey
> 1/2 cup water, as needed

To make cake, place carrot pulp in a large bowl.

Next, process sunflower seeds into a fine powder in your food processor. Slowly add in dates and mix well. Scoop into bowl with carrot pulp. Add nutmeg and cinnamon and mix well.

To make frosting, place cashews, lemon juice, agave, and water in your blender. Blend into a smooth frosting.

Mold dough into desired cake shape.

Spread frosting over cake and serve.

Will keep for four days in the fridge.

FOR 24 SERVINGS, PER SERVING: calories 200, protein 5g, carbohydrates 19g, fat 9g, sugar 11g
PERCENT DAILY VALUES: potassium 10%, vitamin A 55%, vitamin C 4%, calcium 4%, iron 10%, vitamin E 28%, thiamin 19%, riboflavin 4%, niacin 5%, vitamin B6 8%, folate 10%, pantothenic acid 10%, vitamin K 9%, phosphorus 15%, magnesium 18%, zinc 8%, copper 23%, manganese 28%, selenium 12%, dietary fiber 17%

THE REAL CHEEZECAKE

MAKES ONE CAKE

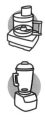

I'm using agave in the cheeze filling to keep it white in color. Feel free to use ¾ cup pitted dates instead if you'd prefer keeping it truly raw. Just make sure to add an extra ½ cup of water as needed to help blend up the dates.
Top with Raspberry Sauce (page 233), or Carob Sauce (page 232).

CRUST

- 1 ½ cups macadamia nuts
- ½ teaspoon sea salt
- ½ cup pitted dates
- ¼ cup shredded coconut

FILLING

- 3 cups cashews
- ¾ cup lemon juice, from about 6 lemons
- ¾ cup agave syrup or honey
- ¾ cup coconut oil
- 1 vanilla bean
- ½ cup water, as needed

To make crust, process the macadamia nuts into small pieces with salt in the food processor. Slowly add dates and mix well.

"Flour" the bottom of a 9-inch springform pan with the shredded coconut. Press crust evenly onto the bottom of the pan. Set aside.

To make filling, blend cashews, lemon juice, agave, coconut oil, and vanilla in your blender. Add just enough water to blend into a smooth kream. Pour into springform pan, and place in the freezer until firm.

Before serving, take cake out of the freezer and remove from the pan while frozen. Place cake on a plate and defrost in the refrigerator for an hour before serving.

Will keep in fridge for five days, and in freezer for more than a week.

FOR 24 SERVINGS, PER SERVING: calories 249, protein 4g, carbohydrates 17g, fat 19g, sugar 11g
PERCENT DAILY VALUES: potassium 5%, vitamin C 6%, calcium 2%, iron 8%, vitamin E 1%, thiamin 7%, riboflavin 3%, niacin 3%, vitamin B6 4%, folate 4%, pantothenic acid 3%, vitamin K 8%, phosphorus 10%, magnesium 14%, zinc 7%, copper 22%, manganese 21%, selenium 4%, dietary fiber 6%

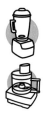

FLORIDA ORANGE-SPICE BARS

MAKES 12 BARS

SYRUP

1 cup pitted dates
1 medium orange, peeled and seeded
½ cup water, as needed

CRUST

1 cup oat groats
2 cups pecans, dry
1 teaspoon ground cinnamon
½ teaspoon grated nutmeg

FILLING

1 large orange
2 cups pitted dates, chopped
3 tablespoons filtered water

To make syrup, blend dates and orange until smooth in your food processor or blender, adding water as needed. Set aside.

To make crust, finely grind oat groats with your Vita-Mix blender dry blade or an electric coffee grinder, and sift out any hard bits with a coarse sieve.

Next, coarsely chop pecans in food processor. Add oat flour, cinnamon, and nutmeg. Pulse to mix. Add syrup 1 tablespoon at a time, until mixture holds together.

Lightly oil a 9-inch square pan and press half of the crust into bottom. Save the remaining half to use as topping.

To make filling, zest orange and set aside. Next, peel, remove seeds, and place orange in food processor with dates and zest and puree until smooth. Add water as needed. Spread mixture over crust.

To serve, crumble remaining half of crust over the top. Press mixture down with your hand to compress and smooth top crust. Cut into triangles and serve.

OPTIONAL: Dehydrate several hours at 104º F until the tops of the bars are warm. Serve warm.

Will keep for four days in the fridge.

FOR 12 SERVINGS, PER SERVING: calories 300, protein 6g, carbohydrates 23g, fat 7g, sugar 18g
PERCENT DAILY VALUES: potassium 14%, vitamin A 3%, vitamin C 21%, calcium 4%, iron 10%, vitamin E 5%, thiamin 18%, riboflavin 4%, niacin 4%, vitamin B6 9%, folate 8%, pantothenic acid 6%, vitamin K 2%, phosphorus 15%, magnesium 16%, zinc 10%, copper 20%, manganese 80%, selenium 4%, dietary fiber 30%

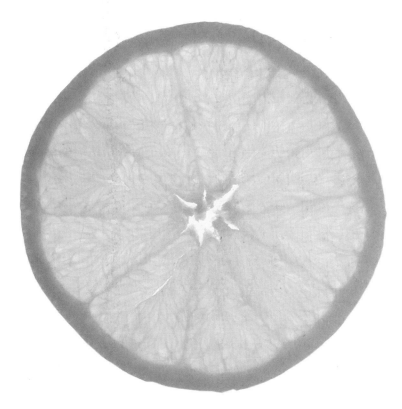

CAROB CRUNCH TORTE

MAKES ONE TORTE

Top with Carob Sauce (page 232) or Raspberry Sauce (page 233)

2 cups almonds, dry
1 teaspoon sea salt
2 vanilla beans, scraped
1 ½ cups pitted dates
¾ cup carob powder
¼ cup Buckwheat Crispies (page 66)

In food processor, chop almonds, salt, and vanilla into small pieces. Slowly add dates and mix well. Empty into mixing bowl with remaining ingredients, and mix well.

To serve, press into an 8 x 9-inch baking pan, or use your hands to roll about ¼ cup at a time into balls.

Will keep for six days in the fridge.

FOR 8 SERVINGS, PER SERVING: calories 311, protein 10g, carbohydrates 32g, fat 14g, sugar 21g
PERCENT DAILY VALUES: potassium 16%, calcium 14%, iron 13%, vitamin E 46%, thiamin 4%, riboflavin 22%, niacin 11%, vitamin B6 8%, folate 6%, pantothenic acid 3%, vitamin K 1%, phosphorus 21%, magnesium 32%, zinc 10%, copper 27%, manganese 53%, selenium 4%, dietary fiber 44%

LEMON COCONUT BARS

MAKES 12 BARS

Serve with Carob Sauce (page 232).

> **1 cup almonds, chopped**
> **1 ½ cups pitted dates (Medjool, khadrawhi, or other semi-soft date)**
> **1 vanilla bean**
> **1 teaspoon sea salt**
> **Zest of 1 lemon**
> **Juice of 1 lemon, about 2 tablespoons**
> **1 cup dried shredded coconut**

In your food processor, chop almonds into small pieces. Use some of this nut powder to "flour" the bottom of a 9-inch square baking pan.

In a mixing bowl, mix remaining ingredients, including the remaining chopped almonds. Press into baking pan.

To serve, chill for a couple hours until firm. Then cut into squares.

Will keep for six days in the fridge.

FOR 12 SERVINGS, PER SERVING: calories 160, protein 4g, carbohydrates 20g, fat 6g, sugar 14g
PERCENT DAILY VALUES: potassium 8%, vitamin C 3%, calcium 4%, iron 6%, vitamin E 15%, thiamin 4%, riboflavin 6%, niacin 4%, vitamin B6 5%, folate 2%, pantothenic acid 2%, phosphorus 8%, magnesium 12%, zinc 4%, copper 10%, manganese 22%, selenium 2%, dietary fiber 17%

DREAMING ABOUT DONUT HOLES

This recipe was inspired by Ede Schweizer, a dear old friend of mine who's also an amazing living foods chef.

You won't be able to eat just one donut. So I recommend tripling this recipe. Donut Holes will keep for over a week in your fridge.

Serve with Berry Compote (page 233).

> 1 ¾ cups almonds
> ½ teaspoon sea salt
> 1 vanilla bean, scraped
> 2 cups dried pineapple, chopped
> 2 cups pitted dates
> ⅓ cup plus ¼ cup shredded coconut

In food processor, place almonds, salt, and vanilla. Process into a fine powder first. Slowly add chopped pineapple and dates, mix well. Place in a large bowl. Mix in ⅓ cup shredded coconut.

To serve, use an ice cream scooper or spoon to form donut holes. Roll holes in ¼ cup shredded coconut.

Will keep for over a week in the fridge.

FOR 24 SERVINGS, PER SERVING: calories 131, protein 6g, carbohydrates 21g, fat 5g, sugar 15g
PERCENT DAILY VALUES: potassium 6%, calcium 3%, iron 3%, vitamin E 13%, thiamin 2%, riboflavin 5%, niacin 3%, vitamin B6 2%, folate 2%, pantothenic acid 1%, vitamin K 1%, phosphorus 6%, magnesium 8%, zinc 3%, copper 7%, manganese 15%, selenium 1%, dietary fiber 11%

icey kreams

LIVING FOODS DOESN'T mean you have to go without frozen treats. When I first started eating raw, there weren't many options for nondairy frozen treats, so I had to invent these raw ice kreams and gelatos to curb my craving for frozen creaminess. I figured all it would take was using a raw nut kream in the same way ice cream uses dairy cream, and it worked! These recipes call for an ice cream maker. If you don't have one, you can instead place your kream into a bowl. Place it in the freezer and stir frequently until frozen.

Make your own sundaes by placing a scoop of ice kream on a piece of Carob Crunch Torte (page 226) with your favorite syrup. Or make a sundae with a banana, scoops of ice kream, and your favorite sauce.

For all ice kream recipes, make sure to use the *least* amount of water possible. This will keep your ice kream smoother, rather than icy.

HAZELNUT GELATO

MAKES 8 SERVINGS

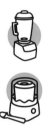

> 1 ½ cups hazelnuts
> 1 ½ cups pitted dates
> Meat of 2 Thai baby coconuts
> 1 vanilla bean
> 3 cups water, use coconut water first, plus other water, as needed

In your blender, blend hazelnuts, dates, coconut meat, vanilla bean, and coconut water first. Use the least amount of liquid possible. Gradually add only as much water as needed for a thick, creamy consistency. Pour into ice cream maker, and chill until frozen.

Will keep for seven days in the freezer. Defrost for 10 minutes before eating.

FOR 8 SERVINGS, PER SERVING: calories 260, protein 6g, carbohydrates 28g, fat 13g, sugar 19g
PERCENT DAILY VALUES: potassium 15%, vitamin C 5%, calcium 5%, iron 10%, vitamin E 30%, thiamin 13%, riboflavin 5%, niacin 5%, vitamin B6 11%, folate 10%, pantothenic acid 4%, vitamin K 6%, phosphorus 11%, magnesium 17%, zinc 6%, copper 28%, manganese 86%, selenium 3%, dietary fiber 22%

VANILLA MACADAMIA ICE KREAM

MAKES 8 SERVINGS

1 vanilla bean
1 ¼ cups macadamia nuts
¾ cup pitted dates
½ cup coconut water
2 cups water, as needed

Blend vanilla bean, nuts, dates, and coconut water until smooth. Add just enough filtered water as needed to create a smooth kream. Put kream into ice cream maker and freeze.

Will keep for seven days in the freezer. Defrost for 10 minutes before eating.

FOR 8 SERVINGS, PER SERVING: calories 199, protein 3g, carbohydrates 14g, fat 13g, sugar 10g
PERCENT DAILY VALUES: potassium 6%, vitamin C 1%, calcium 3%, iron 5%, vitamin E 1%, thiamin 18%, riboflavin 3%, niacin 4%, vitamin B6 4%, folate 1%, pantothenic acid 3%, vitamin K 1%, phosphorus 5%, magnesium 10%, zinc 2%, copper 10%, manganese 46%, selenium 2%, dietary fiber 14%

PUCKERING LEMON MINT ICE

MAKES 8 SERVINGS

Use as a palette cleaner between courses. And top your dessert soups with a scoop before serving.

Juice of 2 lemons, about 4 tablespoons
½ bunch fresh mint leaves, torn into small pieces
1 cup water

Combine lemon juice, mint, and water. Pour into an ice cream maker and freeze.

Will keep for seven days. Defrost for 10 minutes before eating.

FOR 8 SERVINGS, PER SERVING: calories 2, protein 1g, carbohydrates 1g, fat 0g, sugar .2g
PERCENT DAILY VALUES: vitamin A 2%, vitamin C 10%

FRESH APRICOT SORBET

MAKES 8 SERVINGS

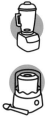

3 cups ripe apricots, peeled, pitted, diced
¼ cup coconut oil
1 vanilla bean
Juice of 1 lime, about 1 tablespoon
½ cup pitted dates
1 cup water, as needed

Blend apricots, coconut oil, vanilla bean, lime juice, and dates. Add only enough water as needed to blend smooth. Pour into your ice cream maker and freeze.

To serve, take sorbet out of the freezer and serve immediately in eight bowls. The coconut oil in this recipe will make your sorbet melt faster. Or store the sorbet in the freezer.

Will keep for seven days in the freezer. Defrost for 10 minutes before eating.

FOR 8 SERVINGS, PER SERVING: calories 230, protein 2g, carbohydrates 24g, fat 12g, sugar 21g
PERCENT DAILY VALUES: potassium 13%, vitamin A 45%, vitamin C 20%, calcium 3%, iron 4%, vitamin E 5%, thiamin 3%, riboflavin 4%, niacin 5%, vitamin B6 5%, folate 4%, pantothenic acid 4%, vitamin K 6%, phosphorus 4%, magnesium 5%, zinc 2%, copper 7%, manganese 7%, dietary fiber 16%

THESE SAUCES ARE a great way to add color and another texture to any dessert. Also see the syrups from the Breakfast of Champions chapter (page 63), like Berry-licious Syrup (page 79), Orange Vanilla Syrup (page 79), Vanilla Syrup (page 79)

CAROB SAUCE

MAKES 8 SERVINGS

> **½ cup pitted dates**
> **1 cup water, plus more as needed**
> **½ cup carob powder**
> **¼ cup extra virgin olive oil**

In your blender, blend dates with water and carob powder until smooth. Add olive oil and more water as needed to make a thick syrup.

Will keep for six days in your fridge.

FOR 8 SERVINGS, PER SERVING: calories 101, protein 1g, carbohydrates 13g, fat 6g, sugar 9g
PERCENT DAILY VALUES: potassium 4%, calcium 3%, iron 2%, vitamin E 4%, thiamin 1%, riboflavin 2%, niacin 1%, vitamin B6 2%, folate 1%, pantothenic acid 1%, vitamin K 5%, phosphorus 1%, magnesium 2%, zinc 1%, copper 3%, manganese 1%, selenium 1%, dietary fiber 14%

RASPBERRY SAUCE

MAKES 8 SERVINGS

It's important to use a food processor, rather than a blender, for this recipe. Otherwise the raspberry seeds will seem like sand.

> **2 cups raspberries**
> **1/2 cup pitted dates**

In your food processor, process raspberries and dates until mixed well.

Will keep for three days in the fridge.

FOR 8 SERVINGS, PER SERVING: calories 43, protein 1g, carbohydrates 11g, fat .2g, sugar 7g
PERCENT DAILY VALUES: potassium 3%, vitamin C 14%, calcium 1%, iron 2%, vitamin E 1%, thiamin 1%, riboflavin 1%, niacin 2%, vitamin B6 2%, folate 2%, pantothenic acid 2%, vitamin K 3%, phosphorus 2%, magnesium 3%, zinc 1%, copper 3%, manganese 12%, selenium 1%, dietary fiber 12%

BERRY COMPOTE

MAKES 8 SERVINGS

> **5 large blackberries or strawberries**
> **1 cup white raisins**
> **Splash of water, as needed**

Blend blackberries and raisins with just enough water as needed to make a thick berry sauce.

Will keep for two days in the fridge.

FOR 8 SERVINGS, PER SERVING: calories 64, protein 1g, carbohydrates 14g, fat .1g, sugar 11g
PERCENT DAILY VALUES: potassium 5%, vitamin C 8%, calcium 1%, iron 2%, vitamin E 1%, riboflavin 2%, niacin 1%, vitamin B6 4%, folate 1%, vitamin K 1%, phosphorus 3%, magnesium 2%, zinc 1%, copper 4%, manganese 5%, dietary fiber 4%

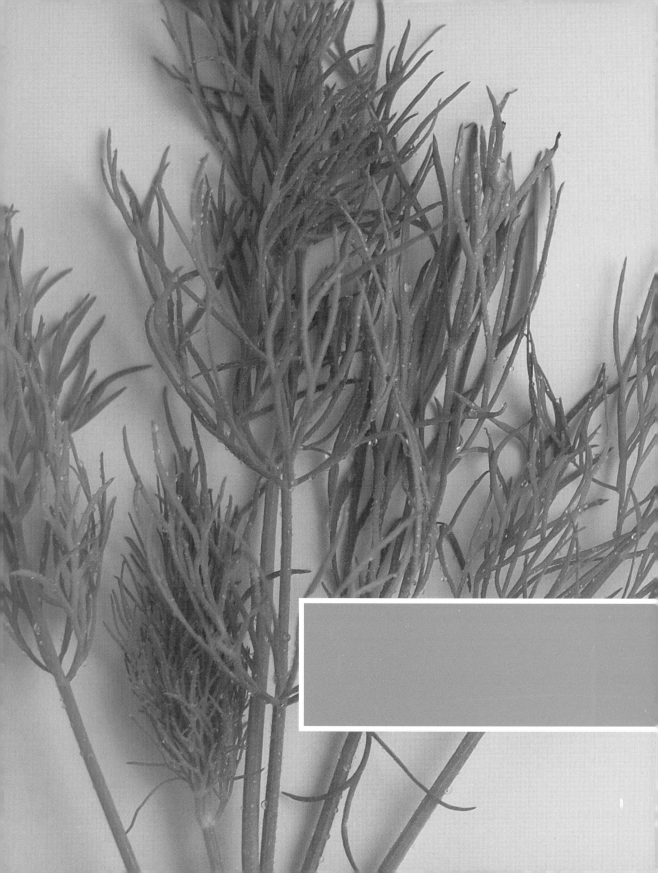

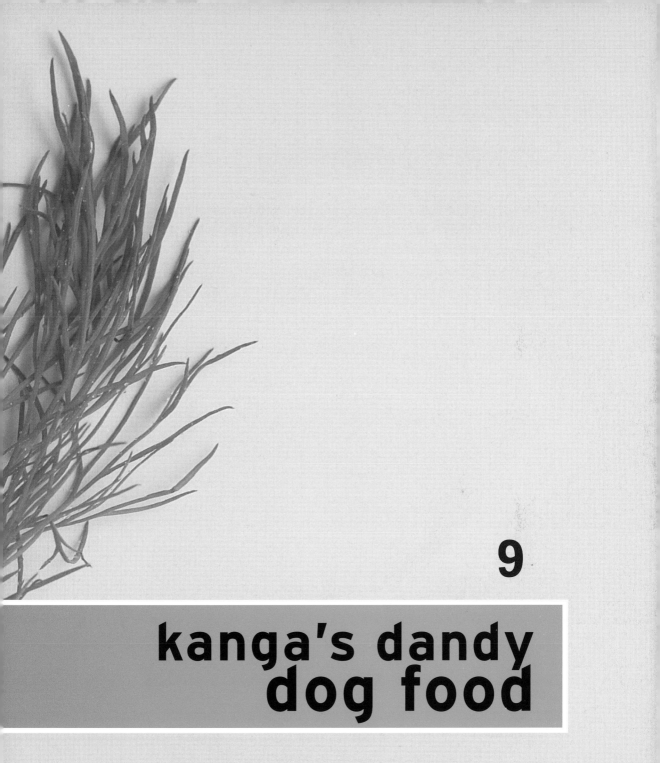

9

kanga's dandy
dog food

dogs love live food!

MY DOG LOVES my vegan organic living cuisine. So do all her dog friends who come to visit. They always rush over to her bowl and lick it clean. At dinners at my house, Kanga's been known to help herself to plates of living cuisine when no one's looking. She eats better than a lot of humans I know. She's a lucky girl.

KANGA'S JOURNEY TO RADIANCE

Kanga is a Rhodesian Ridgeback—a dog that's supposed to be about 90 to 100 pounds. Kanga was very sick when I adopted her. She was about 45 pounds, had kennel cough,

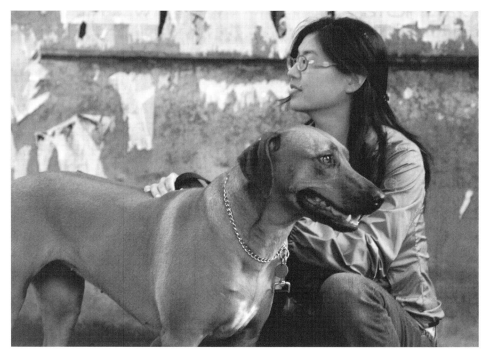

Kanga loves whole fresh food. On her own in nature, that's what she'd be eating.

hung her head low, was depressed, was losing chunks of hair, and was only skin and bone. So I brought her home and started to help her back to health.

Over the next two months, I slowly converted her diet from canned vegetarian dog food to a 100 percent live vegan diet. I made her nut mylks and pâtés, and would mix less and less canned dog food into it over time. I taught her to eat what I did by offering it to her. If she didn't eat it, I'd let her watch me eat it. Then I'd try again, and she'd eat it the next time.

I also learned it's about the shape of the food. Because of the way dogs bite down on food, Kanga likes things to be cut flat. Like apples, I slice them. Round things with skin, like a tomato or grape, took her time to figure out. In the beginning, I'd break open the skin for her. Now she understands to bite down on it.

Within two months, Kanga gained 50 pounds on her vegan living foods diet. Her fur is soft, silky, and super shiny. Other Rhodesian Ridgeback owners stop us and ask to pet her because she's so radiant. They comment on how smooth and soft her fur is compared to their dog.

And for those who may still be skeptical of vegan diets for dogs, our vet in Pennsylvania thinks Kanga's raw vegan diet is great.

FOODS KANGA LOVES

Kanga loves most live foods. And she's got her favorites like avocados, seaweeds, and nuts. But durian is her ultimate favorite, just like her mom.

Durian is a football-size spiny fruit from Southeast Asia. It's a fatty fruit and contains lots of sulfur. So it's really good for you, heals scar tissue, is an aphrodisiac, and makes us release endorphins. Eating durian makes Kanga and me very blissful.

Kanga will do just about anything for durian. We've tailgated many times outside an Asian market, sharing fresh durian in the parking lot. We've hung out in the park in the sun sharing durian. Plus, it made a great treat back when she was in obedience school.

Now that Kanga is in her best health, vibrant, and beautiful, she hops around all the time. This same effect happens for humans, too. When we feel great because our bodies are getting all the nourishment and love it needs, we too become radiant, happy, and bouncy. I've seen this change in many people whom I've consulted for, helping them incorporate more and more fresh organic whole live foods into their diets.

PET FOOD

The fresher and cleaner your pet's food is, the better it is for their bodies, minds, and spirit. Just like for us humans.

Consider all the health problems pets have, like cancer and tumors, for example. Many of these cases can be attributed to the food they're eating. According to the Animal Protection Institute, two-thirds of the pet food made in the United States contains added preservatives. Coloring agents, solvents, oils too rancid or deemed inedible for humans are also used in pet food. The institute reports, "Of the more than 8,600 recognized food additives today, no toxicity information is available for 46% of them."

I don't want to scare you, but if you're interested in finding out more, read "Get the Facts: What's Really in Pet Food" at the Animal Protection Institute Web site: www.api4animals.org.

SAVE THE LIFE OF A PET IN NEED

There're many lovable pets that need homes. Consider adopting an older dog, for example. They can come with many benefits, like already being spayed or neutered, being potty trained and obedience trained, and they are usually calmer and gentler than a younger pup might be.

It's said that pets know and appreciate when you save their life. I guess this is why Kanga is the best dog ever. She's super mellow, always well behaved, and is so easy to share my home and life with. As with all good relationships, my life is better with her around. She's my little angel.

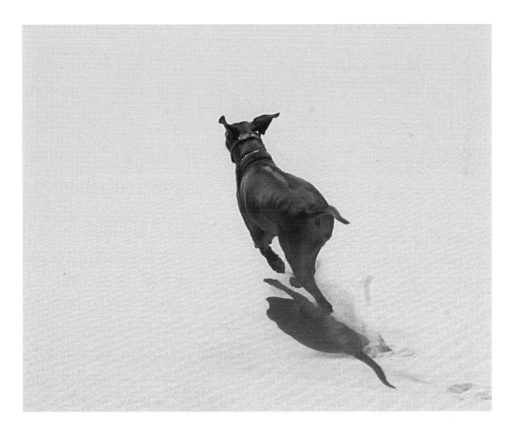

KANGA'S FAVORITE PÂTÉ

Kanga is about 95 pounds and I feed her about 2 cups twice a day. She loves it when I drizzle olive oil over the top of her food before serving. The oil is great for her coat, too, and keeps her sleek and shiny.

All her pooch friends love this pâté, too. They bee-line it over to her food bowl whenever they come to visit, and lick her bowl clean. It's so cute!

1 clove garlic
1 tablespoon sea salt
1 cup sunflower seeds
1 cup almonds, cashews, Brazil nuts, pecans, or walnuts
2 cups greens and vegetables (kale, spinach, squash, carrots)
1 tablespoon fresh herbs (basil, oregano, cilantro, dill)
2 tablespoons extra virgin olive oil

Process garlic and salt into small pieces.. Add sunflower seeds and nuts and process into a powder. Add remaining ingredients and mix well.

To serve, scoop pâté into a dog bowl and drizzle olive oil over the top.

OPTIONAL: Just before serving, I like to mix 1 tablespoon of spirulina blue-green algae or 2 tablespoons of dry wakame into Kanga's food. Dogs love chlorophyll, which is why they eat grass all the time.

GREEN TIP

Kanga Helps Me Reduce My Compost

MAKING DOG FOOD is a great way to use every last morsel of vegetables and herbs.

I use the ends of my zucchini, carrots, and celery, the stems of my kales, collard greens, and herbs in Kanga's food. It's all organic stuff and is made with lots of my love. It gives Kanga her fiber, too.

OUR PETS AND US

Pets are tuned in to how we feel. They know when we're happy or sad, and it affects them, too. I've only ever had dogs, and know they're truly our best friends. Kanga gives me so much unconditional love and support. When I'm super busy, she reminds me to eat, exercise, sleep, and to take a moment to breathe. There've been times when Kanga's made me realize how much stress I was under, because I'd cause her stress.

We owe it to our pets to be happy so they can enjoy being with us. By fueling our bodies and minds with the freshest organic living foods, we're helping ourselves, our families, our pets, and our communities.

KANGA DOG TREATS

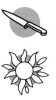

It's important to keep your dog's gums and teeth healthy, especially since they aren't crunching down on dry kibble. These easy-to-make, crunchy treats help remove plaque and freshen dog breath.

Your dog may not be used to these at first. Just like other new foods, you may need to teach him or her how to eat them by taking a bite out of one, then giving it to your pooch to try. Dogs always love what they see us eating!

2 large sweet potatoes, sliced ½-inch thick

Place sweet potatoes on dehydrator trays, and dry at 104º F for twelve hours, or until completely dry.

BLACK SESAME SUNFLOWER DOG BISCUITS

Another crunchy treat dogs love are flax crackers. I like to make them thicker for Kanga, so they clean her teeth as she bites down.

2 batches Black Sesame Sunflower Bread (page 153)

Spread a double batch of bread onto one dehydrator tray and dehydrate seven to eight hours and flip. Use a dog-bone-shaped cookie cutter, or score rectangles into your bread. Dehydrate for another six hours, or until completely dry.

BE YOUR DOG'S BEST FRIEND

Dogs are great stress relievers and are a great excuse for taking time out of your busy day to have fun.

Make time to play, walk, pet, hug, and massage your pooch. It's great to plan social events for your dog, like meeting up with another dog for a hike, or going to the dog park to play with other dogs.

I love seeing Kanga's tail wag, a sign that she's happy.

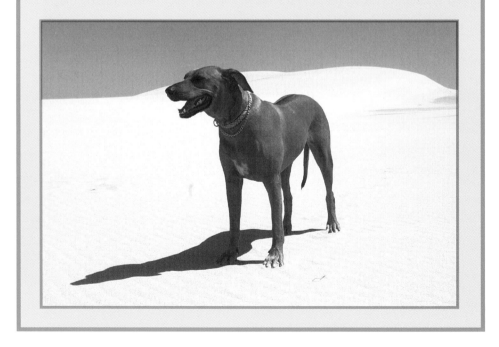

thanks

I'VE SO MANY wonderful people to thank, and can only begin to name a few here.

Thank you to my mother, Jae; brother, Max; and father, Inchol for believing in me and always being there for me. Thank you for teaching me the importance of sharing knowledge with those seeking it, helping people in need, and being responsible for creating the world I want to see around me. Thank you Max, Esq, for countless hours of consulting and master legal advice.

Thank you to three terrific photographers: Ede Schweizer, for your ability to make me look great on film, for sharing all your insights and feedback, and for your dedication to this project from the very start through to this end many years later; Duc Nguyen for eagerly jumping in when you already had an overly full workload to take the most amazing ingredients photos—only you could make a slice of lemon or a sprig of cilantro look so intriguing; and Jim Yeager for stepping up to represent the community lifestyle of Portland, Oregon, with lovely photos of our green city.

Thank you my wonderful SmartMonkey recipe reviewers: Ede Schweizer, Tonya Kay, Teddy Yonenaka, Heather Butler, Ana Sage, and Elena Matsuura; our SmartMonkeys Heather Butler and Kris Dyer for acting as my stylists for our Portland photo shoots; our Southern California SmartMonkey Dawn Ramos for your continued support and invaluable feedback; and a very special thanks to my partner, Peter Wierzbicki, for graciously taking on my workload on top of your already full schedule, and for helping deflect distractions so I could focus on finishing this book.

Thank you to Portland, Oregon: Whole Foods Markets and Steve Gazda, Salud Cooking School Director; Food Front Cooperative Grocery and Holly Jarvis, Dylan Gillis, and Gary Koppen; Deep Roots Farms and Eilif Knutson and Mark Des Marets; and a very special thanks to BodyCote Food Lab's Nidal Kahl and Tim McCann for all your continued support throughout this project, and for gathering all the nutritional panels in lightning speed.

Thank you to Antonio Sanchez for the wonderful icon illustrations.

Thank you to the Northern California crew: Judy Maier's Home and Garden Design and Accessories; and Kevin Garnica and Matt Bolen's Surf 41 Shop in Santa Cruz.

Much gratitude to Renée Sedliar, my editor, and Matthew Lore, our publisher, for believing in this book, and for your commitment to making it great while keeping it real and accessible to many people.

Thank you to Brendan Brazier, Matt Amsden, Lisa Ekus, and Jane Falla for sharing your wisdom with me.

A very special thanks to my dear friend Juliano, who brought live foods to the gourmet platform from which chefs like myself could launch.

ABOUT THE PHOTOGRAPHER

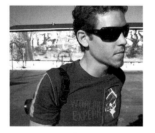

I was compelled to capture this photo of Ede Schweizer, the man behind the camera. His amazing photographs of me in California and my food light up the pages of this book. A live-food enthusiast for many years, his creative vision and positive outlook on life are contagious. Check out more of his travel photography at: www.DecibelDragon.com.

index

NOTE: Page numbers in *italics* indicate recipes that utilize extra portions.

A

accompaniment and side recipes, 137–55
acorn squash
    Mexican Squash "Rice," 142
    in Mushroom Risotto, 188
agave syrup, 30, 39
air pollution, 160
All-American Apple Pie, 211
almond butter
    Almond Kaffir Sauce, 186–87
    shopping for, 28, 186
    in Thai Dipping Sauce, 178
    in Yum Yum Mylk, 57
almonds
    Almond Cinnamon Oatmeal, 69
    Almond Nog, 53
    Almond Pie Crust, 211
    Almond Yogurt, 128
    in Cacao Pudding, 73
    Carob Almond Decadence shake, 53
    in Carob Crunch Torte, *217*, 226
    in Cherry Malt, 51
    in Chocolate Mylk, 56
    in Coconut Snow Cake, 220
    in Donut Holes, 228
    in Garden Pâté, 167
    Ginger Almond Nori Roll, 181
    Ginger Almond Pâté, 167
    in Hollandaise Sauce, 193
    in Lemon Coconut Bars, 227
    in Lemon Pudding, 74
    in Love-the-Chicks Pâté, 81
    in Mexico Mylk, 57
    in Mushroom Risotto, 188
    in smoothies, 47–48
    in Strawberry Kream Swirl, 207
    in Summer Berry Cobbler, 214
    in Taco Nut Meat, 154
    in Vanilla Mylk, 55
aloe, 201
alternative-energy-news.info, 110
American Chemical Society, 136
Anaheim Chilies, Stuffed, with Mole Sauce, 192
Angel-Hair Squash Noodles in Sun-Dried Tomato Marinara, 184
Angel-Hair Squash Pasta in Pesto Sauce, 183
animal products, 111, 112, 113–14
Animal Protection Institute, 238
antibacterial soaps, 203
antibiotic resistant marker genes, 44
antiperspirants, 204
apple cider vinegar, 33
apples
    Apple Pie, 211
    in Curry Dressing, 96
    in Good Morning Muesli, 68
appliances, pedal power for, 110
Apricot Sorbet, 231
arugula
    Arugula with Golden Beets and Walnuts in Orange Miso Dressing, 101
    in Evergreen Salad, 97
Asian greens, about, 98
Asian Greens Salad with Super Asian Dressing, 98
Asian Scramble, 83
Asparagus with Cheezy Sauce, 152
autumn foods, 23
Autumn Pumpkin Pie, 218

avocados
    in Carob Pudding, 73
    on Garlic Walnut Soup, 116
    in Italian Herb Collard Wrap, 177
    Rosemary Guacamole, 150
    Spicy Kream of Avocado Soup, 124
    in Super Asian Dressing, 98
    on Sweet Corn Chowder, 122
    on Thailand Tom Kha Gai, 123

B
Baja Cheeze, 164, *189*
Baja Cheeze Burrito with Taco Nut Meat and
    Red Pepper Corn Salsa, 189
balancing meals, 173
bananas
    about, 54
    Banana Raisin Oatmeal, 69
    in Blue-Green Power shake, 54
    in Carob Pudding, 73
    Cashew Banana Mylk, 59
    Cinnamon Banana Buttermylk, 56
    in Coconut Snow Cake, 220
    in Fruit Parfait, 75
    in Hemp Muesli, 68
basil chiffonade, 120
basil leaves
    in Asian Greens Salad, 98
    in Italian Pizza Cheeze, 161
    in Minestrone Soup, 125
    in Pad Thai, 186–87
    in Pistachio Pesto, 150
    on Pizza, 197
    in Sun-Dried Tomato Marinara, 126
    in Thai Salad Mix, 99
    in Thai Spring Rolls, 178
    Tomato Basil Bisque, 120
beans, difficulty digesting, 148
Beautifying Pumpkin Mylk, 58
beauty on the inside, 200–205
beets, in Arugula with Golden Beets and
    Walnuts, 101
bell peppers
    in Garden Scramble, 82
    in Pad Thai, 186–87
    Red Pepper Corn Salsa, 151
Berry-Licious Syrup, 79
bicycle riding, 110
blackberries
    Berry Compote, 233
    Berry-Licious Syrup, 79

    Summer Berry Cobbler, 214
Black Olive Hummus (bean-free), 149
Black Olive Tapenade, 155
Black Pepper Cheeze, 161, *192*
Black Sesame Asian Slaw with Ginger Cashew
    Mayo, 105
Black Sesame Jewel smoothie, 49
Black Sesame Sunflower Bread, *149, 150, 153,
    155, 162–63, 165, 194–95, 197*
Black Sesame Sunflower Croutons, 154
Black Sesame Sunflower Dog Biscuits, 242
blenders, 15, 16
blueberries
    Berry-Licious Syrup, 79
    Blueberry smoothie, 46
    Blueberry Soup with Cashew Kream, 208
    Summer Berry Cobbler, 214
Blue-Green Power shake, 54
body fat, 205
bok choy
    in Asian Greens Salad, 98
    in Asian Scramble, 83
    Black Sesame Asian Slaw, 105
    on Thailand Tom Kha Gai, 123
    in Thai Salad Mix, 99
Bragg Liquid Aminos, 32, 39
Brazil nuts
    in Baja Cheeze, 164
    Brazil-Broccoli Mash, 143, *196*
    Brazilian Carob Shake, 50
    in Carob Cake, 219
    in Creamy Portabello Bisque, 117
    in Heirloom Tomato Gazpacho, 115
    in Peachy Kream, 52
    in Power Dressing, 103
    in Sun-Dried Tomato Cheeze, 162
Bread, Black Sesame Sunflower, 153
breakfast recipes
    butters, 80
    cereals, 66–71
    pancakes and syrups, 77–79
    puddings, 72–76
    scrambles, 81–83
broccoli
    Brazil-Broccoli Mash, 143
    on Kream of Avocado Soup, 124
    on Thailand Tom Kha Gai, 123
Buckwheat Crispies, 66, 68, 71, 75, 226
burdock root, in Ginger Almond Nori Roll, 181
Burrito, Baja Cheeze, with Taco Nut Meat and
    Red Pepper Corn Salsa, 189

butternut squash, in Walnut Cranberry Squash "Rice," 140
butters, recipes for, 80

C

cabbage. See also bok choy
    about, 92, 189
    for Baja Cheeze Burrito, 189
    Cabbage Kale Slaw in Simple Greek Dressing, 94
    in Confetti Salad, 95
    in Spring Herb Rainbow salad, 96
    in Wakame Hemp Power Slaw, 103, 104
cacao. See cocoa/cacao
cake recipes, 219–28
carbon monoxide (CO), 86–87
carob
    about, 33–34, 39
    Brazilian Carob Shake, 50
    Carob Almond Decadence shake, 53
    Carob Crunch Torte, 217, 226
    Carob Fudge syrup, 217
    Carob Pudding, 73
    Carob Sauce, 226, 227, 232
    Carob Strawberry Bliss smoothie, 47
    in Cherry Malt, 51
    Deep Forest Carob Cake with Fudge Frosting, 219
    in Mexico Mylk, 57
    in Mole Sauce, 192
Carrot Cake with Kream Cheeze Frosting, 222
cashew nuts
    in Black Pepper Cheeze, 161
    Cashew Banana Mylk, 59
    Cashew Coconut Pudding, 73
    Cashew Crust, 212, 213
    Cashew Garlic Parmesan Sprinkle, 151
    Cashew Kream, 208, 209
    Cashew Sour Kream and Chives, 147
    in Cheezecake, 223
    Garlic Cashew Aïoli, 127, 182
    Ginger Cashew Mayo, 105
    Indian-spiced Cashews, 144
    in Kream Cheeze Frosting, 222
    in Mission Fig and Pear Tart, 216
    in Oregano Ricotta, 165
    in smoothies, 46
Cauliflower Miso Mash, 143
Celtic sea salt, 31
cereal recipes, 66–71
chard, in Spring Herb Rainbow salad, 96

Cheezecake, 223
cheeze recipes, 160–65
chemicals
    in air, soil, and water, 12
    in antibacterial soaps, 203
    in antiperspirants, 204
    in drinking water, 136
    in factory-farm raised animals, 112
    in fragrances, 204
    in household cleaning products, 158
    in nail polish, 203
    in processed foods, 44–45
cherries
    Cherry Malt, 51
    in Confetti Salad, 95
cherry tomatoes
    in Asian Greens Salad, 98
    in Italian Herb Collard Wrap, 177
    on Kream of Avocado Soup, 124
    on Thailand Tom Kha Gai, 123
chili peppers
    about, 192
    in Pad Thai, 186–87
    Stuffed Anaheim Chilies with Mole Sauce, 192
    Thai Dipping Sauce, 178
    in Thai Spring Rolls, 178
Chinese cabbage. See bok choy
chlorine in tape water, 135–36
chlorophyll, 104
Chocolate-Hazelnut Mylk, 58
Chocolate Mylk, 56
cholesterol and dairy products, 113, 160
cilantro leaves
    in Baja Cheeze, 164
    on Black Sesame Asian Slaw, 105
    on Heirloom Tomato Gazpacho, 115
    in Mexican Squash "Rice," 142
    in Pad Thai, 186–87
    in Red Pepper Corn Salsa, 151
    in Spanish Scramble, 82
    in Spring Herb Rainbow salad, 96
    on Sweet Corn Chowder, 122
    on Thailand Tom Kha Gai, 123
    in Thai Spring Rolls, 178
    in Walnut Cranberry Squash "Rice," 140
cinnamon
    Almond Cinnamon Oatmeal, 69
    in Carrot Cake, 222
    Cinnamon Banana Buttermylk, 56
    in Mexico Mylk, 57

in Mole Sauce, 192
in Orange-Spice Bars, 224–25
in Pecan Chai Pie on Cashew Crust, 212
in Persimmon Pie, 213
in Pumpkin Pie, 218
citrus juicer, 16
cleaning supplies, 158–59
clothing, 90, 114
cobbler and pie recipes, 210–18
cocoa/cacao
about, 33–34, 39
Cacao Pudding, 73
in Chocolate-Hazelnut Mylk, 58
coconut. See also Thai baby coconuts
butter made from, 28, 80
in Carob Cake, 219
in Carrot Cake, 222
Cashew Coconut Pudding, 73
in Cashew Crust, 212
Coconut Breakfast Cakes, 76, 78
Coconut Snow Cake, 220
in Donut Holes, 228
jerky made from, 139
Lemon Coconut Bars, 227
in Mission Fig and Pear Tart, 216
opening and scraping, 139
Strawberry Coconut Shake, 51
Vanilla Coconut Shake, 50
coconut oil as skin moisturizer, 201
coconut water, 37, 43, 136–37
collard leaves
de-stemming, 177
Italian Herb Collard Wrap, 177
for Mediterranean Dolmas, 146
for Save-the-Tuna Wrap, 179
for Thai Spring Rolls, 178
composting, 86, 87
Confetti Salad in Orange-Cucumber Dressing, 95
corn
Polenta with Mushroom Ragout, 190–91
Red Pepper Corn Salsa, 151
Sweet Corn Chowder, 122
cranberries
in Good Morning Muesli, 68
Walnut Cranberry Squash "Rice," 140
Crepe Kream Stack, 76
Croutons, Black Sesame Sunflower, 154
Crushed Red Pepper-Crusted Cheeze Patty, 162
cucumbers
Cucumber-Orange Dressing, 95
in Green Machine juice, 60

on Heirloom Tomato Gazpacho, 115
Orange-Cucumber Dressing, 95
for sunburn and tired eyes, 201
Thai-style Cucumbers, 142
Tzatziki—Cucumbers in Yogurt, 129
Curry Dressing, 96

D
dairy-free mylk and kream, 55
dairy products, high cholesterol from, 113, 160
dates, 29
Deep Forest Carob Cake with Fudge Frosting, 219
Deglet Noor dates, 29
dehydration, signs of, 135
dehydrators and dehydrating foods. See also dried foods
about, 16, 174–75
Black Sesame Sunflower Bread, 144–45, 242
Buckwheat Crispies, 66
Indian-spiced Cashews, 144
Kanga Dog Treats, 241
Salmon Patties, 193
Stuffed Anaheim Chilies, 192
Sun Burgers, 194
sun drying buckwheat groats, 67
dessert, about, 205–6
dessert recipes
cakes, 219–28
dessert soups, 207–9
icey kreams, 229–31
pies and cobblers, 210–18
sweet sauces, 232–33
diet, balancing your, 173
dill, fresh
on Garlic Walnut Soup, 116
in Mediterranean Dolmas, 146
in Spring Herb Rainbow salad, 96
Sunny Dill Cheeze, 164
dog food recipes, 236–42
Dolmas, Mediterranean, 146
Donut Holes, 228
dried foods. See also dehydrators and dehydrating foods
fruits, 29, 67, 68, 73, 95, 227, 228
herbs and spices, 26, 88, 126, 162, 185, 194
drink recipes
juice, 60
mylks, 54–59

shakes, 50–54
smoothies, 46–49

E

EFAs (essential fatty acids), 54, 130, 202
electrolytes, 43, 135
emotional stressors, 171
endurance from green energy, 64
energy
    life force as, 10
    from nutrient-rich foods, 4, 42, 64–65, 206
Environmental Protection Agency (EPA),
  86–87
environmental stressors, 170, 171
enzymes, 8, 10
essential fatty acids (EFAs), 54, 130, 202
essential oils, 204–5
Evergreen Salad in Sunflower Thyme
  Marinade, 97
exercising, water intake during, 135

F

farmers' markets, 18, 21, 24, 44, 86, 90. *See also*
  living foods; local foods; seasonal foods
fats, quality and quantity, 173
Fender Blender, 110
fennel
    in Arugula with Golden Beets and
      Walnuts, 101
    Lemon Fennel Soup, 121
    Shaved Fennel with Blood Oranges,
      Poppy Seeds, and Micro Greens, 93
fermented raw foods, 130
fermenting yogurt, 128
Fettuccini Squash Noodles in Alfredo Sauce,
  182
fiber
    action of water and, 10, 205
    in dates, 29
    in flax seed, 78
    psyllium powder, 74
    in whole fruit, 46, 60
figs, fresh or dried
    in Hemp Muesli, 68
    Mission Fig and Pear Tart, 216
flax seeds
    in Black Sesame Sunflower Bread, 153
    in Good Morning Muesli, 68
    nutrition and fiber in, 54, 78
    shopping for, 28, 32
    in Sun Burgers, 194–95

Florida Orange-Spice Bars, 224–25
focus from green energy, 65
food combining, simplicity and, 2, 12
food processors (kitchen tool), 15, 16
foods. *See also* dried foods; living foods;
  organic foods
    energy from, 4, 42, 64–65, 206
    local, 2–3, 21, 24, 30, 109
    processed, 44–45, 86
    raw, 7, 8, 130
    seasonal, 21, 22–23, 90, 173
    super foods, 35
fragrances, 204
fresh food. *See* living foods
Fruit Parfait, 75
fruits, shopping for, 34. *See also specific fruits*
Fuzzy Navel Con Kream, 209
Fuzzy Navel shake, 52

G

garbage-free living, 87, 109
garbage timelines, 91
Garden Pâté, 167
Garden Scramble, 82
garlic
    deveining, 95
    effect of raw, 25
Garlic Cashew Aïoli, 127, *182*
Garlic Cashew Parmesan Sprinkle, 151
Garlic Walnut Soup, 116
Gazpacho, Heirloom Tomato, 115
genetically engineered (GE) foods, 44
ginger
    in Almond Kaffir Sauce, 186–87
    in Curry Dressing, 96
    in Garden Pâté, 167
    Ginger Almond Nori Roll, 181
    Ginger Almond Pâté, 167, *181*
    Ginger Cashew Mayo, 105
    in Green Machine juice, 60
    in Japanese Miso-Shiitake Soup, 118–19
    in Kaffir Lime Leaf Dressing, 99
    in Orange-Cucumber Dressing, 95
    in Orange Miso Dressing, 101
    in Power Dressing, 103
    in Super Asian Dressing, 98
global warming, 110
goji berries, about, 67
Goji Berry Sunshine Cereal, 67
Greek Dressing, 94
green energy companies, 14

green juices, 60
Green Machine juice, 60
green planet. *See also* farmers' markets; living
 green
    burden from animal products, 113–14
    composting and recycling for, 18, 86,
      87–88
    quality considerations, 17, 42
    reusing clothing, 90
    toxic-free living, 158–60
greens, 92–105. *See also specific greens*

H
Halawy dates, 29
hazelnuts
    Chocolate-Hazelnut Mylk, 58
    Hazelnut Gelato, 229
health on the inside, 170–75, 204
healthy eating tip, 92
heirloom produce, 109, 126
Heirloom Tomato Gazpacho, 115
hemp and hemp seed oil
    about, 54, 68, 202
    in Angel-Hair Squash Pasta in Pesto Sauce,
      183
    Hemp Muesli, 68
hemp nuts
    on Kream of Avocado Soup, 124
    in Wakame Hemp Power Slaw, 103, 104
hemp protein powder
    about, 35
    in Blue-Green Power, 54
Herb-Crusted Cheeze Patty, 163
herbicides and pesticides, 12
herbs and spices. *See also specific herbs* and
  spices
    desteming fresh herbs, 116
    shopping for, 25–26
hijiki, on Black Sesame Asian Slaw, 105
Himalayan salt, 31
Hirsch, Alan, 26–27
honey, 30, 39
Hot Mustard Sauce, 130, *195*
hummus, 148, 149
hydration, importance of, 134–37
hydrocarbons, 170

I
ice cream maker, 16
icey kream recipes, 229–31

icons for kitchen tools, 16
Indian-spiced Cashews, 144
iodized salt versus sea salt, 30–31
Italian Herb Collard Wrap, 177
Italian Pizza Cheeze, 161, *185*, *197*
Italian Rawzania, 185

J
Japanese Miso-Shiitake Soup, 118–19
juice, 60
Juliano's Raw Restaurant (San Francisco),
  4, 5
julienne peeler, 16

K
kaffir lime leaves
    about, 99
    Almond Kaffir Sauce, 186–87
    Kaffir Lime Leaf Dressing, 99
    in Thai Dipping Sauce, 178
    in Thailand Tom Kha Gai, 123
kale
    Cabbage Kale Slaw, 94
    in Confetti Salad, 95
    in Evergreen Salad, 97
    in Wakame Hemp Power Slaw, 103, 104
Kanga's Dog Treats, 241
Kanga's Favorite Pâté, 240
kitchen tools, 15–16
Kream Cheeze Frosting, 222

L
legumes, difficulty digesting, 148
Lemon Coconut Bars, 227
Lemon Fennel Soup, 121
Lemon Pudding, 74
lemon rinds, cleaning with, 158–59
limes. *See also* kaffir lime leaves
    in Almond Kaffir Sauce, 186–87
    in Apricot Sorbet, 231
    in Kream of Avocado Soup, 124
    in Pistachio Pesto, 150
    in Power Dressing, 103
living foods. *See also* energy; local foods;
  organic foods; seasonal foods
    about, 8, 9, 44
    Ani's path to, 3–7, 113
    bananas, 54
    berries, 214
    dates, 29

desserts made from, 205
energy from, 4, 42, 64–65, 206
enzymes, 8, 10
fermented raw foods, 130
flax seed, 78
fresh water in, 134
herbs and spices, 25
nuts and seeds, 27
olives, 32
sea salt, 31
sea vegetables, 104
uncooking and, 109
vanilla beans, 27
living green. *See also* green planet
balancing meals, 173–75
beauty on the inside, 200–205
earth-friendly fashions, 114
green energy, 64–65
the joy of uncooking, 108–14
organic, local, bulk foods for, 86–91
quality over quantity, 42–45
stress reduction, 170–72
toxic-free, 158–60
in urban environment, 14
water and, 134–37
Living Tree Community Foods (Berkeley, CA),
   32
local businesses, shopping at, 89–90
local foods, 2–3, 21, 24, 30, 109. *See also*
   farmers' markets; seasonal foods
Love-the-Chicks Pâté, 81, *82*, 83

M

macadamia nuts
   in Cheezecake crust, 223
   in Italian Pizza Cheeze, 161
   in Nacho Cheeze, 165
   Vanilla Macadamia Ice Kream, 230
maca powder, 35
Madagascar vanilla beans, 27
Made in Mexico Mylk, 57
main dish recipes
   knockoffs, 189–97
   pastas, 182–88
   wraps and rolls, 176–81
malnutrition, 44
mandoline slicer, 16
Mango Cobbler, 215
Mango Lassi smoothie, 47
maple syrup, USDA grade B, 30, 39

Mediterranean Dolmas, 146
Medjool dates, 29
mental clarity from green energy, 64
Mexican Squash "Rice," 142
Mexico Mylk, 57
micro greens
   about, 93
   Shaved Fennel with Blood Oranges, Poppy
      Seeds, and Micro Greens, 93
mindfulness, 10
Minestrone Soup, 125
mint leaves
   Lemon Mint Ice, 230
   in Pad Thai, 186–87
   in Thai Salad Mix, 99
   in Thai Spring Rolls, 178
miso, unpasteurized
   about, 31
   Cauliflower Miso Mash, 143
   Japanese Miso-Shiitake Soup, 118–19
   Miso Gravy, 127
   Orange Miso Dressing, 101
Mission Fig and Pear Tart, 216
mizuna, in Asian Greens Salad, 98
MooShoes.com, 114
muesli, 68
mung bean sprouts
   in Black Sesame Asian Slaw, 105
   in Ginger Almond Nori Roll, 181
   in Pad Thai, 186–87
   in Thai Salad Mix, 99
   in Thai Spring Rolls, 178
Mushroom Gravy, 190, *196*
Mushroom Ragout, Polenta with, 190–91
Mushroom Risotto with White Truffle-infused
   Olive Oil, 188
mushrooms, marinating, 110
mustard greens, in Evergreen Salad, 97
Mustard Seed Dressing, 100
mylk recipes, 54–59

N

Nacho Cheeze, 165
nail polish, 203
Nama Shoyu, 31, 39
National Cancer Institute, 29
natural fibers, 159
natural food stores, 18
nitrogen oxides, 170
nori, 176

nut and seed butters, 28
nutritional stressors, 171–72
nuts and seeds. See also specific types of nuts
   and seeds
      shopping for, 27–28, 32, 186
      soaking, 38, 72

O

oat groats
      Almond Cinnamon Oatmeal, 69
      Banana Raisin Oatmeal, 69
      in Orange-Spice Bars, 224–25
      SmartMonkey Bar Oatmeal, 71
oils, shopping for, 32
Olive Butter, 80
olives
      Black Olive Hummus, 149
      Black Olive Tapenade, 155
      in Italian Rawzania, 185
      on Pizza, 197
      shopping for, 32
onions, marinating, 100
oranges
      in Apple Pie, 211
      Fuzzy Navel, 52
      Fuzzy Navel Con Kream, 209
      in Miso Gravy, 127
      in Mission Fig and Pear Tart, 216
      Orange-Cucumber Dressing, 95
      Orange Miso Dressing, 101
      Orange-Spice Bars, 224–25
      Orange Vanilla Syrup, 79
      in Pecan Chai Pie on Cashew Crust, 212
      in Shaved Fennel with Blood Oranges,
         Poppy Seeds, and Micro Greens, 93
oregano leaves
      in Italian Herb Collard Wrap, 177
      in Italian Rawzania, 185
      in Minestrone Soup, 125
      Oregano Ricotta, 165
      on Pizza, 197
organic farms, 44
organic foods. See also living foods
      beautiful skin from, 200
      benefits to our planet, 86–91
      at farmers' markets, 18, 21, 24, 44, 86, 90
      as investment in preventive care, 17, 86
      nutrient density of, 10, 12, 42
      selecting, 20
organic self-care products, 159, 200–202
oxygen in uncooked food, 8

P

Pad Thai Noodles in Almond Kaffir Sauce,
   186–87
pancakes and syrups, 77–80
pasta and noodle recipes, 182–88
pâté recipes, 81, 166–67
peaches
      in Fruit Parfait, 75
      in Good Morning Muesli, 68
      Peachy Kream shake, 52
pears
      in Mission Fig and Pear Tart, 216
      Pear Frosty smoothie, 48
pecans
      in Coconut Snow Cake, 220
      in Fuzzy Navel, 52
      in Mango Cobbler, 215
      in Orange-Spice Bars, 224–25
      Pecan Chai Pie on Cashew Crust, 212
      in Praline Mylk, 59
      Spinach Salad with Persimmons and
         Spiced Pecans, 102
      Sweet Spiced Pecans, 102, 145
      in Vanilla Coconut Shake, 50
pedal power appliances, 110
persimmons
      about, 102
      Persimmon Pie, 213
      Spinach Salad with Persimmons and
         Spiced Pecans, 102
pesticides and herbicides, 12
Pesto, Pistachio, 150
pets and their humans, 239, 241, 242
physical stressors, 171, 206
pie and cobbler recipes, 210–18
Piña Colada smoothie, 48
pineapple
      in donut holes, 228
      in Piña Colada smoothie, 48
pine nuts
      in Coconut Snow Cake, 220
      in Mediterranean Dolmas, 146
      in Ricotta Cheeze, 163
Pistachio Pesto, 150, 183
Pizza with Sun-Dried Tomatoes, Black Olives,
   and Fresh Italian Herbs, 197
plastic water bottles, 37
Polenta with Mushroom Ragout, 190–91
Portabello Bisque, Creamy, 117
Portabello Steak, Marinated, and Brazil-
   Broccoli Mash with Mushroom Gravy, 196

Portland, Oregon, 6, 7
Power Dressing (salad), 103, 104
Praline Mylk, 59
prep time, 3
preventive care, 17
processed foods, 44–45, 86
produce, heirloom, 109
productivity from green energy, 65
psyllium powder
    about, 74
    in Cauliflower Miso Mash, 143
    in Lemon Pudding, 74
pudding recipes, 72–76
Pumpkin Pie, 218
pumpkin seeds
    in Good Morning Muesli, 68
    in Pumpkin Mylk, 58
    in Pumpkin Pie, 218
    in Summer Berry Cobbler, 214

R

raisins
    in Garden Pâté, 167
    Raisin Banana Oatmeal, 69
Raspberry Sauce, 226, 233
raw food, 7, 8, 130
recipes, utilizing the, 36–40
recycling, 87–88, 90
Red Pepper Corn Salsa, 151, *189*
Red Pepper-Crusted Cheeze Patty, 162
renewable energy options, 14
Ricotta Cheeze, 163, 165
ripe foods, 20
romaine lettuce, for Save-the-Tuna Roll, 180
rosemary
    in Black Olive Tapenade, 155
    in Herb-Crusted Cheeze Patty, 163
    in Italian Herb Collard Wrap, 177
    in Kream of Avocado Soup, 124
    in Portabello Steak, 196
    Rosemary Guacamole, 150
    in Spring Herb Rainbow salad, 96

S

salad and salad dressing recipes, 92–105
"Salmon" Patties with Hollandaise Sauce, 193
salt, sea, 30–31
sandwich wraps, 176–81
sauce and dip recipes
    Alfredo Sauce, 182
    Almond Kaffir Sauce, 186, 187
    Almond Yogurt, 128
    Cheezy Sauce, 152
    Garlic Cashew Aïoli, 127
    Hollandaise Sauce, 193
    Hot Mustard Sauce, 130
    Miso Gravy, 127
    Mole Sauce, 192
    Mushroom Gravy, 190, *196*
    Pesto Sauce, 183
    Sun-Dried Tomato Catsup, 129
    Sun-Dried Tomato Marinara, 126
    Thai Dipping Sauce, 178
    Tzatziki—Cucumbers in Yogurt, 129
Save-the-Salmon Patties with Hollandaise
    Sauce, 193
Save-the-Tuna Pâté, 166, *179, 180*
Save-the-Tuna Roll, 180
Save-the-Tuna Wrap, 179
scrambles, recipes for, 81–83
sea salt, 30–31
seasonal foods, 21, 22–23, 90, 173. *See also*
    living foods; local foods
sea vegetables, 33, 103, 104, 176
seeds. *See* nuts and seeds; *specific seeds*
sesame seeds. *See also* tahini
    in Asian Scramble, 83
    Black Sesame Asian Slaw, 105
    Black Sesame Jewel smoothie, 49
    Black Sesame Sunflower Bread, *149, 150,*
        153, 155, 162–63, 165, 194–95, 197
    Black Sesame Sunflower Croutons, 154
    Black Sesame Sunflower Dog Biscuits, 242
    in Good Morning Muesli, 68
    in Super Asian Dressing, 98
shakes, recipes for, 50–54
Shallot Lemon Dressing, 102
Shaved Fennel with Blood Oranges, Poppy
    Seeds, and Micro Greens, 93
shiitake mushrooms
    in Asian Scramble, 83
    Japanese Miso-Shiitake Soup, 118–19
shopping
    buying in bulk, 89
    at farmers' markets, 18, 21, 24, 44, 86, 90
    local products, 89–90
    for produce, 34
    at supermarkets, 24
shopping checklist
    apple cider vinegar, 33
    carob and cocoa/cacao, 33–34
    dried fruits, 29

fruits and vegetables, 34
herbs and spices, 25–26
nuts and seeds, 27–28, 32, 186
oils, 32
olives, 32
salts, 30–32
sea vegetables, 33
super foods, 35
sweeteners, 29–30
vanilla beans or vanilla extract, 26–27, 39
sides and accompaniment recipes, 137–55
simplicity, 2
SmartMonkey Bar Cereal, 71
SmartMonkey Bar Oatmeal, 71
SmartMonkey Foods, 4–7, 14, 70–71, 206
smoothie recipes, 43, 46–49
soup recipes, 115–25
Sour Kream and Chives, 147
soy sauce, unpasteurized and unheated, 31, 39
Spanish Scramble, 82
spices. See herbs and spices
spinach
    in Angel-Hair Squash Pasta in Pesto Sauce, 183
    in Baja Cheeze Burrito, 189
    in Evergreen Salad, 97
    in Garden Scramble, 82
    in Ginger Almond Nori Roll, 181
    in Green Machine juice, 60
    on Kream of Avocado Soup, 124
    in Spanish Scramble, 82
    Spinach Salad with Persimmons and
        Spiced Pecans in Shallot Lemon
        Dressing, 102
    in Thai Salad Mix, 99
    Wilted Spinach Salad with Marinated
        Onions in Mustard Seed Dressing, 100
spiralizer, 16, 182
spirulina
    about, 35
    in Blue-Green Power, 54
spring foods, 23
Spring Herb Rainbow in Kreamy Curry
    Dressing, 96
Spring Rolls with Dipping Sauce, Thai, 178
squash, peeling, 140
stainless steel water bottles, 37, 43
stamina from green energy, 64
stoves, health hazards from, 109
strawberries
    Berry Compote, 233
    Berry-Licious Syrup, 79

Strawberry Carob Bliss smoothie, 47
Strawberry Coconut Shake, 51
Strawberry Kream Swirl, 207
    for sunburn, 201
stress, controlling or eliminating, 170–71, 206
Stress Solution, The (Miller and Smith), 170
Stuffed Anaheim Chilies with Mole Sauce, 192
substitutions, 39
Summer Berry Cobbler, 214
summer foods, 23
sunblock, 202
Sun Burgers on Black Sesame Sunflower Bread
    with Sun-Dried Tomato Catsup, 192
sun-dried tomatoes
    in Italian Herb Collard Wrap, 177
    in Italian Rawzania, 185
    in Mediterranean Dolmas, 146
    in Minestrone Soup, 125
    Sun-Dried Tomato Catsup, 129, 195
    Sun-Dried Tomato Cheeze, 162
    Sun-Dried Tomato Hummus (bean-free),
        148
    Sun-dried Tomato Marinara, 126, 184, 185, 197
sun drying, 67
sunflower seeds
    in Black Olive Hummus, 149
    in Black Sesame Sunflower Bread, 153
    in Carrot Cake, 222
    in Cheezy Sauce, 152
    in Hemp Muesli, 68
    in Love-the-Chicks Pâté, 81
    in Save-the-Tuna Pâté, 166
    shopping for, 27
    in SmartMonkey Bar Cereal, 71
    Sun Burgers, 194–95
    Sunflower Thyme Marinade, 97
    Sunny Dill Cheeze, 164, 177, 193
Super Asian Dressing, 98
super foods, 35
supermarkets, 24
Sweet Corn Chowder, 122
sweeteners, 29–30, 39
sweet sauce recipes, 232–33
Sweet Spiced Pecans, 102, 145
syrup recipes, 79

T
Taco Nut Meat, 154, 189
tahini
    in Black Olive Hummus, 149
    Chocolate-Hazelnut Mylk, 58

shopping for, 28
    in Sun-Dried Tomato Hummus, 148
    in Yum Yum Mylk, 57
tat soi, in Asian Greens Salad, 98
tea tree oil, 203–4
Thai baby coconuts. See also coconut
    in Carob Almond Decadence (opt.), 53
    Coconut Chutney, 138
    Coconut Kream Pie with Carob Fudge on
      Brownie Crust, 217
    electrolytes in, 37, 135
    in Hazelnut Gelato, 229
    opening and scraping, 139
    in Pad Thai, 186–87
    in Piña Colada (opt.), 48
    in Strawberry Coconut Shake (opt.), 51
    in Vanilla Coconut Shake (opt.), 50
Thailand Tom Kha Gai, 123
Thai Salad Mix with Kaffir Lime Leaf Dressing, 99
Thai Spring Rolls with Dipping Sauce, 178
Thai-style Cucumbers, 142
thyme leaves
    in Black Olive Tapenade, 155
    on Creamy Portabello Bisque, 117
    in Garlic Cashew Aïoli, 127
    in Italian Rawzania, 185
    on Polenta with Mushroom Ragout, 190–91
    Sunflower Thyme Marinade, 97
Tomato Basil Bisque, 120
Tom Kha Gai, Thailand, 123
toxic-free living, 158–60
tumeric
    in Cheezy Sauce, 152
    in Love-the-Chicks Pâté, 81
    in Nacho Cheeze, 165
"Tuna" Pâté, 166, 179, 180
"Tuna" Roll, 180
"Tuna" Wrap, 179
Tzatziki—Cucumbers in Yogurt, 129

U

uncooking as art form, 108–12
U.S. National Pollutant Emission Estimates
  report, 170

V

vanilla beans
    deseeding, 49
    shopping for, 26–27, 39
Vanilla Coconut Shake, 50
Vanilla Macadamia Ice Kream, 230

Vanilla Mylk, 55
Vanilla Orange Syrup, 79
Vanilla Syrup, 79
vegan fashion, 114
vegan uncooking, 111–12
vegetable juicer, 16
vegetables, shopping for, 34. See also specific
  vegetables
Vegetarian Society, 113
Vita-Mix blenders, 15
volatile organic compounds (VOCs), 158, 170

W

wakame, 103
Wakame Hemp Power Slaw, 103, 104
walnuts
    Arugula with Golden Beets and Walnuts,
      101
    Garlic Walnut Soup, 116
    in Ricotta Cheeze, 163
    in smoothies, 49
    in Sweet Corn Chowder, 122
    in Taco Nut Meat, 154
    Walnut Cranberry Squash "Rice," 140
water, 10, 134–37, 173
watercress, in Asian Greens Salad, 98
water filtration systems, 136
weight loss, 205
winter foods, 23
wire whisk, 16
wrap and roll recipes, 176–81

Y

Yum Yum Mylk, 57

Z

zucchini
    in Angel-Hair Squash Noodles in Sun-Dried
      Tomato Marinara, 184
    in Angel-Hair Squash Pasta in Pesto Sauce,
      183
    in Black Olive Hummus, 149
    Fettuccini Squash Noodles in Alfredo
      Sauce, 182
    in Italian Rawzania, 185
    in Minestrone Soup, 125
    in Pad Thai, 186–87
    in Sun-Dried Tomato Hummus, 148
    in Thai Spring Rolls, 178

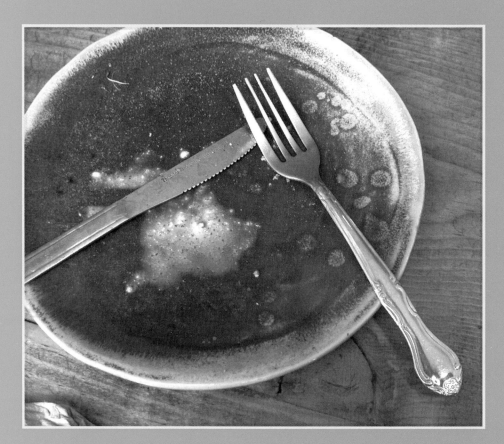

Yum.

Eat up ecstatic culinary delights and boost your radiant health. May our children's children enjoy all the beauty of our green planet. Let's keep striving to outdo ourselves each and every day. Chow down, and get your green on!